More Case Prese...
Paediatric Anaesth...   ...Care

More Case Presentations in Paediatric Anaesthesia and Intensive Care

Neil S. Morton MBChB FRCA FRCPCH
Consultant in Paediatric Anaesthesia, Department of Anaesthesia,
Royal Hospital for Sick Children, Yorkhill NHS Trust, Glasgow, UK
Senior Lecturer, University of Glasgow, UK

Edward I. Doyle MD FRCA
Consultant in Paediatric Anaesthesia, Department of Anaesthesia,
Royal Hospital for Sick Children, Edinburgh, UK

Jane Peutrell MBBS FRCPEd FRCA
Consultant in Paediatric Anaesthesia, Department of Anaesthesia,
Royal Hospital for Sick Children, Yorkhill NHS Trust, Glasgow, UK

Ros Lawson MBChB FRCA
Consultant in Paediatric Anaesthesia, Department of Anaesthesia,
Royal Hospital for Sick Children, Yorkhill NHS Trust, Glasgow, UK

Pam Cupples MBChB FRCA
Specialist Registrar in Paediatric Anaesthesia, Department of
Anaesthesia, Royal Hospital for Sick Children, Yorkhill NHS Trust,
Glasgow, UK

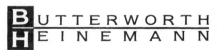

OXFORD AUCKLAND BOSTON JOHANNESBURG MELBOURNE NEW DELHI

Butterworth-Heinemann
Linacre House, Jordan Hill, Oxford OX2 8DP
225 Wildwood Avenue, Woburn, MA 01801-2041
A division of Reed Educational and Professional Publishing Ltd

 A member of the Reed Elsevier plc group

First published 2000

©Reed Educational and Professional Publishing Ltd 2000

British Library Cataloguing in Publication Data
A catalogue record for this book is available from the British Library

Library of Congress Cataloguing in Publication Data
A catalogue record for this book is available from the Library of Congress

ISBN 0 7506 4215 7

Typeset by BC Typesetting, Keynsham, Bristol BS31 1NZ
Printed and bound in Great Britain by Biddles Ltd, Guildford and King's Lynn

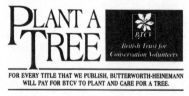

To our parents and to our patients

Contents

Preface

Trainees and specialists in anaesthesia, intensive care and emergency medicine who occasionally have to look after children may not have a clear plan for dealing with problem paediatric cases. Common problems encountered daily by the specialist paediatric anaesthetist or intensivist may be rarities for the general anaesthetist or intensivist. The discussion of cases in advance is helpful, and the aim of this book is to use illustrative case scenarios to emphasize the safe, modern approach to a wide variety of problems in the fields of paediatric anaesthesia and intensive care. Key references are provided for further reading. Paediatric intensive care is developing as a specialty in its own right, and this book shows the scope of current practice. We hope the format of the book will allow it to be used for self study and tutorial discussion by trainees but also to provide continuing medical education for established senior staff.

N. S. Morton, E. I. Doyle, J. Peutrell, R. Lawson and
P. Cupples, Glasgow

Case presentations, questions and answers

Case 1

You are called to review a 5-year-old boy on the paediatric oncology ward who is undergoing treatment for acute lymphoblastic leukaemia. The child has just completed an intensive course of chemotherapy and radiotherapy in preparation for bone marrow transplantation. He has developed severe ulceration of his mouth and is having difficulty in eating and drinking due to the pain. He is also experiencing dyspepsia and profuse diarrhoea.

Questions

1. What is the most likely diagnosis, and what complications may arise?
2. What is your approach to the pain management of this child?

Answers

1. The child is showing classic signs and symptoms of acute mucositis. This is an acutely painful syndrome involving the mucosa of the oral cavity and pharynx. Mucositis commonly extends to involve the other gastrointestinal mucosal surfaces, especially the oesophagus.

   Inflammation and ulceration of the mucous membranes is caused by the local effects of radiotherapy and chemotherapy, which damage the rapidly dividing cells of the epithelial lining of the mouth and the whole gastrointestinal tract. This impairs its barrier function, producing pain and inflammation lasting several weeks.

The pain is severe, constant and burning in nature, and is exacerbated by drinking, eating and talking. If the lower gastrointestinal tract is involved then a colorectal mucositis may develop producing severe rectal pain, tenesmus, diarrhoea, mucus discharge and bleeding.

Complications that may arise are dehydration and malnutrition due to poor oral intake, and patients are also at increased risk of secondary infections. The most common secondary infections are with *Candida albicans* and, in the neutropenic patient in particular, *Herpes simplex*.

2. Pain management is delivered by three main routes; topically, enterally or parenterally. Antifungal and antiviral agents are also used as appropriate.

Topical preparations

Diphenhydramine hydrochloride is an antihistamine with mild analgesic properties, which is used locally to soothe the painful buccal mucosa. If significant amounts are swallowed it may cause drowsiness. A formulation is available that includes *kaopectin*, which helps the diphenhydramine to adhere to the mucosal surface and thus makes systemic absorption less likely.

Choline salicylate gel (Bonjela) has mild analgesic actions; however, there is the risk of salicylate poisoning if this formulation is used too frequently.

Benzydamine hydrochloride (Difflam) is a NSAID that is absorbed through the skin and the mucosa. It also has mild local anaesthetic actions, and can be used as a gargle or as a spray. Problems may arise due to a stinging sensation on application.

Corticosteroids such as dissolved betamethasone tablets can be used as a gargle.

Local anaesthetic preparations include 2% lignocaine viscous gel and benzocaine spray.

Enteral preparations

Antacids include:

- Sodium bicarbonate – problems may arise with belching due to carbon dioxide production and alkalosis with prolonged use.
- Hydrogen peroxide – an oxidizing agent with a direct cleansing effect.

Mucosal coating agents include:

- Sucralfate – a complex of aluminium hydroxide and sulphated sucrose. This works by adhering to the mucosa and protecting it from the acid/pepsin attack.
- Mucosal adhesive film – this uses grade M hydroxypropyl cellulose, ethanol, tetracaine, thiamphenicol and triacetin. This formulation makes a 0.1-mm film over the oral mucosa, giving pain relief for 4–6 hours.

Parenteral preparations

Intravenous opiates are required due to the extreme nature of the pain. Morphine can be given by continuous infusion or via a patient-controlled analgesia regimen (Table 1.1). The doses of narcotics required are invariably high, and it has been found that PCA regimens produce less sedation and the morphine requirements are lower than when a continuous infusion is used. These patients are invariably receiving anti-emetic prophylaxis to cover the effects of their chemotherapy. Tolerance may develop if PCA is needed for a number of weeks, but a self-weaning regimen can be programmed into the device by lengthening lockout intervals and reducing the bolus dose size (Table 1.2). In general, a reduction of total daily morphine consumption of around 20 per cent per day is well accepted in the resolution phase of mucositis.

Table 1.1 Patient-controlled analgesia (PCA) regimen for mucositis

Initial titrated loading dose 0.1–0.2 mg/kg by slow i.v. injection, repeated until comfort attained

PCA bolus dose 20–40 μg/kg, lockout interval 5 minutes, background infusion rate zero

Larger doses than average may be needed.

Table 1.2 Weaning programme

- Maintain same bolus dose initially
- Gradually increase lockout interval from 5 to 20 minutes over a number of days
- Reduce bolus dose
- Aim for approximately 20 per cent reduction in daily morphine consumption per 24 hours

Antifungal and antiviral agents

Nystatin and clotrimazole are required for treatment of secondary infection with *Candida*.

Acyclovir is required in the neutropenic patient at risk of secondary infection with *Herpes simplex*.

Key learning points

- Mucositis is an extremely painful complication of chemo-therapy.
- Opioids in large daily doses are often needed for pain control over a period of weeks.
- PCA is the best delivery method if the child is able to use the device.
- Self-weaning is readily achievable using simple adjustments to lockout intervals and bolus doses.

Further reading

MORTON, N. S. (1998). *Acute Paediatric Pain Management. A Practical Guide.* W. B. Saunders.

Case 2

A 9-year-old boy is scheduled to undergo bilateral otoplasty. His parents are worried that he may be teased when he moves on to senior school, and have requested the surgery. He, however, does not seem affected by having moderately prominent ears, and does not wish to have an operation.

Questions

1. How do you approach the situation when arriving to assess the boy preoperatively?
2. What would be the legal standpoint in this case?

Answers

1. It is important to listen to the opinions of all the people concerned in the decision-making process and establish the facts before deciding the final outcome. An assessment of the relationship between the boy and his parents should be made, and it may be desirable to interview the boy on his own to allow him to express his views more fully. The parents' reasons for requesting surgery should be ascertained and explained to their son. There is all too often a tendency to assume that a parent knows what is best for their child and that they should assume responsibility for consent to a procedure being undertaken. When attempting to obtain informed consent, the information has to be imparted to the child as well as his parents in such a way as to ensure the child's full comprehension of the risks and benefits as far as that is possible. It should be borne in mind that this is a purely cosmetic operation and not a medical requirement.
2. The legal age of consent for medical, surgical or dental treatment is 16 years or over. However, under both English and Scottish law there exists the facility for a child aged less than 16 years to consent (or otherwise) to a procedure, providing they are deemed competent to do so by the medical practitioner attending the child. This came about as a result of the Gillick case in England in 1985 ('Gillick competence'), and the Age of Legal Capacity (Scotland) Act 1991.

Assessing competence to consent is often complex and sometimes contentious. The three ways of testing are:

a. *Status* – does the patient belong to a group usually assumed to be incompetent, such as a very young child?
b. *Outcome* – is the decision competent such that it is likely to result in a desirable outcome?
c. *Function* – can the patient pass tests of general ability, either to decide about the particular operation, or to show general competence?

A competent child should be able to understand the nature, purpose and possible consequences of the proposed treatment, as well as the consequences of non-treatment.

If the child is judged competent, it is the child's consent alone that is legally effective, and parents lose any right they may have had to consent on the child's behalf.

The issue of 'best interest' arises if, for example, a child refused consent to emergency surgery such as an appendicectomy. In England, a person with parental responsibility or the court may authorize treatment that is in the child's best interests.

Under Scottish law it may be that the competency of the child in the individual case needs to be assessed carefully, and legal advice may have to be sought.

If the 9-year-old boy is of sufficient maturity to have understood the information presented to him and has had the time to consider it, then his refusal to consent should be respected and is legally binding. It may be that as he gets older he requests the surgery himself, but it should be left to him to decide.

Key learning points

- For elective surgery in a competent child, the child's consent is paramount.

Further reading

ALDERSON, P. (1993). *Children's Consent to Surgery*. Open University Press.
GMC (1999). *Seeking Patients' Consent: The Ethical Considerations*. GMC.
THE MEDICAL DEFENCE UNION (1997). *Consent to Treatment*. Medical Defence Union Ltd.

Case 3

A 6-year-old girl with severe spastic diplegia is having a femoral osteotomy.

Questions

1. What is cerebral palsy?
2. Discuss the anaesthetic implications of the condition.
3. What are the options for postoperative analgesia?

Answers

1. Cerebral palsy is an abnormality of posture and movement caused by brain injury occurring before 2 years of age. The commonest causes are prematurity, and low birth weight. Others causes include: hypoxia or trauma during delivery; pre-natal infections (e.g. rubella or cytomegalovirus); congenital malformations of the brain (e.g. agenesis of the corpus callo-sum); meningitis; brain tumour or its treatment (i.e. radiation or surgery); intracranial haemorrhage; and some genetic conditions. Cerebral palsy is non-progressive, but skeletal deformity worsens as the effects of muscle imbalance become more pronounced with age.

   Cerebral palsy is classified according to the physiological effects on the nervous system ('physiological classification'), the distribution of limb involvement ('anatomical classifica-tion'), or the ability of the child to walk:

Physiological classification

a. *Pyramidal type*: Damage to the cerebral cortex usually pro-duces spasticity. These children have 'clasp-knife' rigidity and increased reflexes. They frequently develop contractures and bony deformities.
b. *Extra-pyramidal type*: Damage to the basal ganglia or cere-bellum tends to produce athetosis or ataxia.

Pyramidal and extrapyramidal cerebral palsy often co-exist.

Anatomical classification

Anatomical patterns of presentation include hemiplegia (one side of the body), diplegia (a symmetrical pattern with the legs affected more than arms), or paraplegia (legs only). Quadriplegia affects the whole body, including the cranial nerves, and is often asso-ciated with severe learning difficulties.

2. Children who have developed contractures, deformity of bones or instability of joints may need surgery (e.g. rotational osteotomy of the femur, arthrodeses or lengthening of ten-dons) to limit or correct the deformity and allow mobilization or better posture in a wheelchair. Cerebral palsy affects many systems of the body, and can have major implications for anaesthesia.

Nervous system

Children with cerebral palsy may have severe intellectual impairment. They can also be of normal intelligence but have problems communicating with others (e.g. because of sight or hearing impairment, or the inability to articulate clearly). It is important to prepare them carefully before surgery so they are clear about what is happening and, for older children, to ensure that they have given informed consent.

Epilepsy is a common association, and epileptogenic drugs such as enflurane or methohexitone should be avoided. Unexpected bleeding during surgery has been reported in patients treated for epilepsy with valproic acid. Valproic acid may impair coagulation by several mechanisms, including inducing thrombocytopenia or platelet antibodies, or decreasing fibrinogen concentration.

Some children will have ventriculo-peritoneal shunts to treat neonatal hydrocephalus secondary to intraventricular haemorrhage. If the shunt is functioning normally and the patient has no clinical features of raised intracranial pressure, no specific precautions are necessary and prophylactic antibiotics are not routinely given.

Ventilatory system

Kyphoscoliosis occurs in 60 per cent of children with spastic quadriplegia (see DeLuca, 1996). The effects can be difficult to assess because these children may not be able to cooperate with pulmonary function tests.

Gastrointestinal system

Gastro-oesophageal reflux is common and is associated with poor nutrition, recurrent chest infections and the risk of pulmonary aspiration of gastric contents during anaesthesia.

Children with cranial nerve weakness and difficulty in swallowing may have a problem with drooling of saliva. Atropine (20 μg/kg orally) may be useful premedication to reduce oropharyngeal secretions.

Locomotor system

Generalized deformity of the joints and bones can cause difficulties in positioning the child for surgery. Excessive uncontrolled movement may make intravenous cannulation before the induction of anaesthesia difficult.

Children with severe spasticity often take medication to reduce muscle tone. Baclofen inhibits transmission at a spinal level and depresses the central nervous system, but can produce excessive sedation and hypotonia. Diazepam may also produce excessive sedation. Dantrolene acts directly on skeletal muscle and is probably the drug of choice for spasticity because it has few side effects.

In contrast to upper motor neurone lesions acquired later, suxamethonium does not induce hyperkalaemia in children with cerebral palsy. The response to non-depolarizing muscle relaxants is variable; some children are sensitive and others resistant. Resistance may result from concomitant use of anti-epileptic medication (see Martyn *et al.*, 1992). Because of the unpredictable response, neuromuscular block should be monitored during anaesthesia.

3. Pain after hip surgery in children with cerebral palsy has two components: that associated directly with surgery, which can be controlled with analgesics (e.g. systemic opioids, epidural analgesia, peripheral nerve blocks or simple analgesics); and muscle spasm, which is treated by reducing muscle tone (e.g. with benzodiazepines or epidural analgesia). Children having a femoral osteotomy usually require postoperative analgesia for 2–3 days.

Opioids

Morphine is the commonest opioid used for pain relief after major surgery in children. It gives analgesia but no muscle relaxation, and spasm may be a problem. You should not prescribe intramuscular injections in children because they are painful unless delivered through an indwelling cannula (e.g. into the deltoid muscle). After major operations, morphine is best delivered either by continuous infusion or by patient- or nurse-controlled analgesia (PCA or NCA) systems. Intermittent injections of morphine given by nurses are associated with poor control of pain because concentrations of morphine fluctuate widely.

Continuous infusions produce better pain relief compared with intermittent injections without increasing the side effects. A loading dose of morphine 75–100 μg/kg followed by a continuous infusion of 10–40 μg/kg per hour is a suitable scheme. If morphine 1 mg/kg body weight is added to 50 ml of diluent, an infusion of 1 ml/hour delivers 20 μg/kg per hour.

Patient-controlled analgesia has the major advantages that the child will not operate the control button if over sedated, and delivery of morphine is titrated to the child's needs. Most authors describe PCA using morphine delivered intravenously, and recommend a bolus dose of 20 μg/kg with a lockout interval of 5–15 minutes initially (see Gillespie and Morton, 1992). You may need to adjust the settings; a percentage of successful demands persistently less than 60 per cent would indicate too low a rate of morphine delivery. In contrast to adults, a background infusion during the first postoperative night is associated with a more constant rate of morphine delivery, better patterns of sleep and probably superior analgesia. A suitable rate of background infusion is 2–8 μg/kg per hour.

PCA can also be delivered subcutaneously, and this may have advantages compared with the intravenous route (i.e. a lower rate of morphine consumption, a greater proportion of valid demands and fewer episodes of hypoxia).

Patient-controlled analgesia systems have been used in children as young as 4 or 5 years of age. The suitability of the technique will depend upon the child's ability to understand the concept and their physical ability to operate the hand set. A PCA system may be less useful to children with intellectual impairment or severe movement disorders. NCA is an alternative technique in which nurses can operate the control button according to a strict protocol (Table 3.1). Most schemes use a background infusion of up to 20 μg/kg per hour and a lockout interval of 30 minutes (see Lawson, 1998).

The commonest side effects from morphine delivered by PCA, NCA or continuous infusion are nausea, vomiting, constipation and itching (Gillespie and Morton, 1992). The main danger is respiratory depression caused by an idiosyncratic sensitivity to morphine by the child or failure of the system (drug or programming error by the operator; malfunction of the pump; reflux of opioid along infusion tubing or 'siphoning'). You should either

Table 3.1 Guidelines for nurse-controlled analgesia (Lawson, 1998)

Pump activation:
- pain score 'moderate or severe'
- request from patient

Contraindications to pump activation:
- pain score 'asleep, nil or mild'
- sedation score 'unrousable'
- breathing rate < 12 per minute in a child older than 5 years, or < 20 per minute in a child younger than 5 years
- oxygen saturation less than 94 per cent breathing room air

Table 3.2 Monitoring and hourly recording of child receiving PCA using morphine

SpO₂

Breathing rate

Sedation score – eyes open:
- spontaneously = 0
- to speech = 1
- to shake = 2
- unrousable = 3; CALL DOCTOR

Pain score:
- no pain = 0
- asleep = A
- not really sore = 1 ($\equiv$ mild pain)
- quite sore = 2 ($\equiv$ moderate pain)
- very sore/crying = 3; CALL DOCTOR ($\equiv$ severe pain)

Nausea score:
- none = 0
- nausea only = 1
- ×1 vomit in last hour = 2
- > 1 vomit in last hour = 3; CALL DOCTOR

Number of successful demands and number of total demands

use a dedicated cannula for the opioid infusion or an anti-reflux valve if it is to run along with an intravenous infusion. To prevent gravity free-flow of the contents of the syringe into the patient, the delivery system should be no more than 80 cm above the child and the syringe should be connected through an anti-siphon valve.

A monitoring protocol has been developed for children receiving PCA (Table 3.2), assessing the rate of breathing, oxygen saturation whilst breathing air, sedation, pain and nausea. This scheme can be modified for children given continuous infusions of opioids (i.v., s.c. or epidural) or NCA. In patients breathing air, pulse oximetry is a sensitive indicator of depressed ventilation.

Extradural analgesia
Extradural analgesia provides pain relief and muscle relaxation, and may inhibit the muscle spasm common after orthopaedic operations in children with cerebral palsy. Single injection techniques into the caudal or lumbar epidural space are less appropriate because of the need for prolonged postoperative analgesia. Most practitioners insert a lumbar catheter and prescribe a continuous infusion or repeated injections of local anaesthetic.

Table 3.3 Suggested schemes for epidural analgesia in children having operations on the legs

1. Initial volume of 0.25% bupivacaine of 0.75 ml/kg (children < 20 kg) or 0.1 ml/cm (children > 100 cm in height).

2. Initial volume of 0.25% bupivacaine of 0.5 ml/kg and a subsequent infusion of 0.08 ml/kg per hour.

The doses used are empirical, because there is no reliable formula to predict the extent of block (see Rowney and Doyle, 1998). Suitable schemes for orthopaedic surgery are given in Table 3.3. Further doses can be injected according to clinical response but the loading dose of bupivacaine should not exceed 2–2.5 mg/kg with a maximum of 0.5 mg/kg/hour thereafter to prevent toxic side effects. (In neonates and young infants use half these doses.)

Technical problems (patchy blocks; leakage from the puncture site; occlusion or disconnection of the catheter) can lead to the loss of up to 17 per cent of epidurals and a need for intensive support from the pain service. These problems are associated principally with the use of catheters with a small diameter (0.63 mm), and have been reduced with the introduction of a kit for children containing an 18-G Tuohy needle and a catheter of 0.9 mm diameter. The larger catheter is also potentially safer because you cannot reliably aspirate blood or cerebrospinal fluid through a 0.63-mm diameter catheter lying within a vessel or the subarachnoid space.

Epidural analgesia in children has an excellent record of safety, and serious complications are rare. Hypotension associated with epidural analgesia is uncommon in children younger than 6–8 years who are not hypovolaemic. Systemic toxicity from local anaesthetics is uncommon if the dose is kept within accepted recommendations, unless the child has other risk factors (e.g. reduced clearance because of hepatic resection; idiopathic epilepsy; or febrile convulsions) (see Peutrell and Mather, 1996). Migration of catheters into the subarachnoid space and excessively high blocks are unusual, and these complications may be detected by regularly assessing the height of the block and the child's ability to move the legs. Pressure areas should be regularly inspected.

The addition of opioids improves the quality of analgesia; minimizes the dose and side effects of local anaesthetics; and provides some sedation, which may be beneficial in younger children (see Rowney and Doyle, 1998). Appropriate doses are given in Table 3.4. An alternative approach is to use only local anaesthetic

Table 3.4 Suggested doses of opioids for postoperative epidural analgesia in children (Rowney and Doyle, 1998)

Opioid	Dose
Fentanyl	0.1–0.5 μg/kg per hour
Diamorphine	25–50 μg/kg bolus and 5–50 μg/kg per hour
Morphine	30–75 μg/kg bolus and 5 μg/kg per hour

solutions in the epidural space, and prescribe intravenous opioids in small doses (e.g. morphine 25–50 μg/kg) to be given if required. Common side effects of epidural opioids include nausea and vomiting, and itching. The relative contribution of opioid and local anaesthetic to the incidence of urinary retention is uncertain because both probably play a part. Many of these minor side effects can be treated with small doses of intravenous naloxone (1–5 μg/kg per hour).

Ventilatory depression is a very rare in children older than 12 months but is potentially serious. The scheme given for monitoring of children receiving PCA can be modified to detect this.

Nerve blocks and wound infiltration
The hip joint is supplied by the femoral, obturator and sciatic nerves, and the skin at the site of incision by the lateral cutaneous nerve of the thigh (below the greater trochanter) and the sub-costal nerve (above the greater trochanter). You can block the main components of sensation (the femoral, obturator and lateral cutaneous nerves of the thigh) using a fascia iliaca compartment block. The block can be extended into the postoperative period by inserting a catheter into the compartment. The major disadvantage is that the technique will not include the subcostal nerve and the articular branch of the sciatic nerve. Although local anaesthetic can be infiltrated into the proximal wound and block the sciatic nerve, these 'single injection' techniques will not provide sufficient duration of postoperative analgesia.

Simple analgesics
Non-steroidal analgesic drugs have an opioid sparing effect in children, with a reduction of opioid requirements of up to 40 per cent. Paracetamol given in adequate dose may have a similar effect. Appropriate schemes are given in Table 3.5.

14

Table 3.5 Suggested doses of paracetamol and some non-steroidal analgesic drugs in children

Paracetamol (maximum of 90 mg/kg during first 24 hours)
1. Loading dose of 20 mg/kg orally and 15 mg/kg 4-hourly
2. Loading dose of 30–40 mg/kg rectally and 20 mg/kg 6-hourly

Non-steroidal anti-inflammatory drugs
1. Diclofenac 3 mg/kg per day in two or three divided doses orally or rectally
2. Ibuprofen 5 mg/kg orally 6-hourly

Benzodiazepines

Intermittent muscle spasm is a major component of pain in children with cerebral palsy after hip surgery, and also worsens the pain of incision. Benzodiazepines in low dose (e.g. diazepam 0.1 mg/kg every 6 hours, or midazolam 10–30 μg/kg per hour) are helpful and do not produce excessive sedation. These doses are considerably lower than those used for sedation, but the sedative and respiratory depressant effects of benzodiazepines are additive with opioids and these children should be monitored carefully to detect ventilatory depression.

Key learning points

- Multimodal analgesia is effective in the majority of children.
- Epidural analgesia is recommended where muscle spasm is likely to be a problem.
- Low dose benzodiazepines are effective in managing muscle spasm.

Further reading

DeLUCA, P. A. (1996). The musculoskeletal management of children with cerebral palsy. *Ped. Clin. North Am.*, **43**, 1135–50.

GILLESPIE, J. A. and MORTON, N. S. (1992). Patient-controlled analgesia for children: a review. *Paed. Anaesth.*, **2**, 51–9.

LAWSON, R. A. (1998). Opioid techniques. In: *Acute Pediatric Pain Management. A Practical Guide* (N. S. Morton, ed), Ch. 6, pp. 127–69. W. B. Saunders.

MARTYN, J. A. J., WHITE, D. A., GRONERT, G. A. *et al.* (1992). Up- and down-regulation of skeletal muscle acetylcholine receptors effects on neuromuscular blockers. *Anesthesiology*, **76**, 822–43.

PEUTRELL, J. M. and MATHER, S. J. (1996). *Regional Anaesthesia for Babies and Children*. Oxford University Press.

ROWNEY, D. A. and DOYLE, E. (1998). Epidural and subarachnoid blockade in children. *Anaesthesia*, **53**, 980–1001.

Case 4

An 11-year-old boy with severe learning difficulties presents on the dental list for extractions and conservation management. He is known to have an abscess requiring treatment. On arrival in the anaesthetic room he is resistant to attempts to get him to lie on the trolley and is shouting that he wants to go home, flailing all his limbs wildly. He weighs 70 kg, and requires two male care assistants to look after him.

Questions

1. What are the options for anaesthetic management at this point?
2. What are the issues of consent in this case?
3. Outline some possible techniques of anaesthesia for dental examination in the child with severe learning difficulties.

Answers

1. The first aim is to ensure that neither the patient nor any assistant is harmed whilst struggling in the anaesthetic room. This may be difficult, as the frightened boy may be very strong and difficult to control. As it is usually fear of the unknown that is producing this reaction, it may be possible to calm the situation by one of the carers known to him explaining what is going to happen. Often by this stage, however, no reasoning is possible. It is then necessary to establish the urgency of the procedure and whether it may be possible for the boy to return later after improved preoperative preparation and pre-medication. It is extremely unlikely that his dental abscess is life-threatening, and therefore the most sensible (and humane) course of action is to postpone surgery. On the rare occasion that postponement is not possible, intramuscular ketamine (up to 10 mg/kg) has been used to induce anaesthesia in an urgent situation.
2. In the case of a child with learning difficulties, consent can be given by either parents or nominated carers in charge. Although an 11-year-old child with normal learning ability may be able to give consent (or otherwise) if deemed 'competent' by the medical practitioner, this is obviously not

pertinent in this case. If the boy's parents are not in attendance, then it is the person who holds the Residence Order or any other court order in relation to the child who has the right to consent on the child's behalf.

3. Various anaesthetic induction and maintenance techniques have been described for use in dental anaesthesia for children with severe learning difficulties, but often patients will not let anyone near them. Therefore it is the preparation and premedication of such patients that should perhaps receive greatest attention. Oral premedication is often the easiest to administer, particularly if there has been a relatively prolonged fasting time and the agent is disguised in a drink such as orange juice. *Ketamine*, in a dose of 10 mg/kg orally, has been used successfully in many such cases. It takes around 30 minutes to have full effect and then allows anaesthetic induction with relative ease. As expected, increased oral and endobronchial secretions have been documented and, if given in a higher dose than 10 mg/kg, excitatory effects have become distressing. Recovery time in a darkened environment to minimize emergence delirium takes around 4–6 hours. This is a potential disadvantage in day-case patients. However, it is still usually easier to manage such patients in a day-case environment to minimize disruption to the daily routine and decrease further disorientation. The use of an antisialogogue is recommended.

Midazolam is also useful as a premedicant, although it gives a shorter 'window of opportunity' in which to perform an anaesthetic induction. It can be given orally in a dose of 0.5 mg/kg (maximum 15 mg) mixed with a flavoured drink (~20 ml) or paracetamol elixir to disguise the bitter taste of the intravenous formulation. A cherry-flavoured formulation is available in some countries. Midazolam takes effect in 30 minutes, but usually only lasts for around 20 minutes. Midazolam can also be administered by the intranasal route and transmucosally in the mouth. When given intranasally, a dose of 0.2 mg/kg has been used with marked improvement in the behavioural patterns of previously combative patients. Nasal administration can be distressing for children, and can produce a burning sensation in the nose. Occasionally midazolam produces increased patient distress and disorientation. An important adjunct to premedication is the use of topical local anaesthesia prior to venous cannulation, but again in this patient group even the application of EMLA cream may become an impossible task. After premedication this is often easier, and the use of amethocaine gel may be more acceptable in some cases as it looks different (patients may identify EMLA with previously failed venous access attempts) and acts within 30 minutes. The choice of maintenance technique is probably not as important for the successful procedure as the choice of premedication and patient preparation. Some centres employ clinical child psychologists to assist in this preparation, although this may not be practical in the child with an urgent problem.

Key learning points

- In cases where patients are unable to give their consent, judgement about the urgency of the surgical procedure and the implications of not proceeding must guide therapy.
- Restraint is neither safe nor acceptable in such situations; however, holding the child to protect him from injury is acceptable. Parental involvement can be very helpful. Preparation of the child to allay fears and pharmacological premedication are also important.
- Oral midazolam is the preferred agent for premedication.

Further reading

ANTILA, H., VALLI, J., VALTONEN, M. and KANTO, J. (1992). Comparison of propofol infusion and isoflurane for maintenance of anesthesia for dentistry in mentally retarded patients. *Anesth. Prog.*, **39(3),** 83–6.

FUKATU, O., BRAHAM, R. L., YANASE, H. *et al.* (1993). The sedative effects of intranasal midazolam administration in the dental treatment of patients with mental disabilities. Part 1. The effect of a 0.2 mg/kg dose. *J. Clin. Ped. Dent.*, **17(4),** 231–7.

PETROS, A. J. (1991). Oral ketamine. Its use for mentally retarded adults requiring day care dental treatment. *Anaesthesia*, **46,** 646–7.

Case 5

A 4-year-old boy with the diagnosis of epidermolysis bullosa is admitted for release of skin contractures of his left hand. On examination he is small for his age with areas of moderate blistering on his trunk, and he has had several hospital admissions due to skin infections in the past.

18

Questions

1. What are the main features of epidermolysis bullosa?
2. What are the anaesthetic implications of the disease?
3. What special precautions should be taken in preparing the anaesthetic room and child prior to surgery?
4. What might be a suitable anaesthetic technique for the case?

Answers

1. Epidermolysis bullosa (EB) is a heterogeneous mix of rare, inherited diseases, characterized by separation of the epidermis and/or dermis following shear forces on the skin or mucosa. This results in the formation of mucocutaneous bullae over all areas of the body. The condition can be divided into scarring and non-scarring forms. The scarring commonly occurs with the recessive form of EB dystrophica and often affects the extremities, with fusion of digits. In addition, the mouth, tongue and oesophagus can be involved with microstomia, ankyloglossia and oesophageal stricture formation. Teeth can be severely dysplastic, and laryngotracheal involvement has been reported.

   Patients may present with severe blistering after minor trauma, which can lead to scarring and deformity with chronic infection, potential malnutrition and sepsis.

   With improved management regimens over recent years, survival into adulthood is common.
2. Complications of EB requiring surgery are now more frequent due to the improved survival of these patients. Thus children may present for orthopaedic and plastic surgery, or require dental work. The over-riding anaesthetic consideration is the prevention of any type of shear force or indeed any trauma to the skin and mucosal surfaces. This greatly influences the care with which the child is positioned and the degree and type of monitoring utilized. Preoperatively, there is the potential risk of poor nutrition, anaemia and dehydration plus concomitant infection. There is the possibility of a difficult airway due to microstomia and poor dentition. Laryngeal stenosis has been reported in a few EB patients who had not been intubated previously. Airway instrumentation carries the risk of causing oral mucosal blistering and potential laryngotracheal damage with intubation. However, it appears from

a number of studies that intratracheal lesions are not produced in the scarring form of EB provided a well-lubricated under-sized endotracheal tube is used. Intravenous access may be problematic due to previous scarring and deformity, as may the performance of peripheral nerve blockade.

3. It is important that all the equipment and monitoring apparatus is appropriately sized and lubricated prior to the arrival of the child in the anaesthetic room. The operating table should be covered with a soft mattress and particular care taken to cover all pressure points on the patient with lubricated gauze. Facemasks and laryngoscopes can be covered with petroleum jelly or hydrocortisone ointment. Oral airways should be avoided if possible. Endotracheal tubes several sizes smaller than calculated should be available and well lubricated.

   The use of adhesive tape or stickers is contraindicated, and poses a considerable problem with regard to conventional monitoring. A pulse oximeter probe can be used if all adhesive is covered barring the light-emitting diode and photodiode. ECG electrodes can be used with care if just the central gel area is positioned for the patient to lie on. If deemed necessary, the blood pressure cuff can be applied with soft padding beneath it.

   Intravenous access may require securing with a suture. It is also obviously important to avoid a struggling child at induction by use of appropriate premedication and parental presence if possible.

4. The aims of the anaesthetic technique are to avoid any sort of skin and mucosal trauma whilst keeping the patient still and comfortable postoperatively. Both general anaesthetic and regional techniques with sedation have been utilized for patients with EB. In this case the child requires analgesia of his left arm for a reasonably short procedure, and therefore the use of a brachial plexus block along with i.v. ketamine (0.5–1 mg/kg) incrementally could be used. This technique has been used successfully in a 4-year-old girl, with great care being taken when performing the block using the axillary approach and a nerve stimulator. This necessitated the placement of a ground electrode, which was connected to a saline-soaked sponge placed under the patient's back. The use of ketamine minimized the potential for instrumentation of the airway being required, although full resuscitation equipment should always be prepared.

Key learning points

- Minimal contact and instrumentation are the main principles of anaesthetic management.
- Avoid adhesive contacts with the skin.

Further reading

FARBER, N. E., TODD, J., TROSHYNSKI, M. D. *et al.* (1995). Spinal anesthesia in an infant with Epidermolysis Bullosa. *Anesthesiology*, **83**, 1364–7.

HOLZMAN, R. S., WORTHEN, H. M. and JOHNSON, K. L. (1987). Anaesthesia for children with junctional epidermolysis bullosa (letalis). *Can. J. Anaesth.*, **34(4)**, 395–9.

KAPLAN, R. and STRAUCH, B. (1987). Regional anesthesia in a child with Epidermolysis Bullosa. *Anesthesiology*, **67**, 262–4.

Case 6

You are called to the accident department to help resuscitate a new-born baby with an abdominal wall defect and external herniation of the bowels. The baby was born at home to a teen-aged mother who had concealed the pregnancy.

Questions

1. What is the differential diagnosis? Briefly describe the abdominal wall defect and associated abnormalities.
2. Summarize the major preoperative problems and important points of resuscitation.
3. What surgical techniques of closure are commonly used? How would you anaesthetize this baby for surgery? What intra- and immediate postoperative problems might you anticipate?

Answers

1. The diagnosis in this baby is either exomphalos (omphalocoele) or gastroschisis.

   Exomphalos is a midline defect of the umbilical cord thought to result from failure of the viscera to return to the abdominal cavity during embryological development at 10 weeks gestation. The defect ranges from a few centimetres to the full length of the anterior abdominal wall, but tends to be large (see Paidas et al., 1994). The viscera, usually including the liver, are extruded through the umbilical ring and enclosed within a membranous sac of peritoneum and amnion. The extrusion of most of the viscera limits growth of the abdominal cavity (see Dykes, 1996). The bowels and liver are structurally and functionally normal (see Langer, 1993). Associated congenital anomalies occur in 50–60 per cent of affected foetuses, and include:

a. Chromosomal abnormalities (particularly trisomy 13 and 18) in 10 per cent of live-births
b. Congenital heart disease in 24–35 per cent of live-births
c. Neurological abnormalities (e.g. meningomyelocoele, anencephaly and hydrocephalus) in about a quarter of foetuses
d. Other gastrointestinal anomalies (e.g. malrotation and imperforate anus) and skeletal abnormalities (e.g. arthrogryposis multiplex, limb and vertebral malformations).

Exomphalos can be part of a concurrent syndrome, the most important of which is the Beckwith–Wiedemann syndrome, which affects about 10 per cent of babies with exomphalos. Severe neonatal hypoglycaemia secondary to hyperinsulism is the most significant feature (Engstrom et al., 1988).

The outcome in exomphalos is largely determined by the associated anomalies and chromosome defects. Sixty per cent of foetuses are aborted because of severe associated malformations. About 80 per cent of live-born babies survive (see Dykes, 1996).

In gastroschisis the defect is lateral to the insertion of the umbilicus, usually on the right, and is often small. The bowels lie outside the abdominal cavity and are not enclosed in a membranous sac (see Dykes, 1996). They are often shortened, thickened and damaged, and covered with a fibrous peel (see Langer, 1993). The liver usually remains within the abdomen, which tends to grow to a more normal size sac (see Dykes, 1996). The outcome is largely determined by the condition of the bowel and the complications of surgery and parenteral nutrition. About 90 per cent of affected foetuses survive.

Associated congenital anomalies, excluding those secondary to the bowel pathology, occur in 20 per cent of patients (e.g. chromosome abnormalities, amniotic band syndrome and limb defects). Most abnormalities associated with gastroschisis are secondary to the bowel pathology, and include intestinal atresia, stenosis, ischaemia or perforation, malrotation and volvulus (see Paidas *et al.*, 1994).

Premature birth occurs in a third of babies with either condition. Intrauterine growth retardation affects 37 per cent of those with exomphalos and 60 per cent of those with gastroschisis.

Both conditions are associated with impaired pulmonary function. Functional residual capacity at a mean of 5 months of age is decreased compared with normal babies. Giant exomphalos is particularly associated with pulmonary insufficiency and high mortality rates probably secondary to pulmonary hypoplasia. X-ray examination shows a narrow chest and small lung area.

2. The major preoperative problems of abdominal wall defects in babies are: ventilatory failure with large defects; fluid loss and shock; bowel distension; heat loss and hypothermia; damage to the herniated viscera; and infection (see Langer, 1996). You must also search for and treat any associated significant abnormalities, e.g. Beckwith–Wiedemann syndrome (Engstrom *et al.*, 1988) or congenital cardiac disease. If an antenatal diagnosis is made (i.e. with raised alpha-fetoprotein concentration and positive ultrasound scan), the mother should be transferred before delivery to a regional centre with access to neonatal surgery.

Recognition and treatment of ventilatory insufficiency

Babies with giant exomphalos may have pulmonary hypoplasia and ventilatory insufficiency and need intubation of the trachea and positive pressure ventilation before surgery.

Fluid resuscitation and reducing fluid loss

Gastroschisis is associated with a greater fluid loss through evaporation than exomphalos because the bowels are not enclosed in a membranous sac. Large amounts of fluid may be sequestrated in the bowel lumen in both conditions.

An intravenous cannula should be sited as soon as possible, and adequate volumes of warmed colloid given (bolus of 10 ml/kg initially, and then reassess). The requirement for further volume is assessed by measuring the heart rate (which should be less than 160 beats per minute), the capillary refill time (which should be less than 2 seconds), the core–peripheral temperature gradient and the peripheral oxygen saturation (a poor or absent signal may indicate hypovolaemia). Urine output should be greater than 2 ml/kg per hour. Evaporative losses can be significantly reduced by putting the lower half of the baby, including the herniated viscera, into a sterile polythene bag.

Reducing heat loss and preventing hypothermia
Putting the bowels in a polythene bag reduces heat loss through evaporation and, by decreasing air movement, also reduces convective losses. The aim should be to reduce cold stress and prevent non-shivering thermogenesis by nursing the baby in a thermoneutral environment, either beneath a radiant heater or in an incubator. The heat supplied should be controlled to maintain the temperature of the anterior abdominal wall at 36.5 °C. Core and skin temperatures should be monitored.

Reducing bowel distension
Large volumes of fluid may be sequestered in the bowel lumen in gastroschisis or a large exomphalos. The bowels can be decompressed and the risk of aspiration reduced by passing a nasogastric tube (size 6 or 8 French gauge) and leaving it on free drainage.

The viscera can be protected from damage by enclosing them in a sterile polythene bag, as above. The risk of infection in gastroschisis is high because there is no covering membrane, and antibiotics should be given before surgery.

3. Primary closure is the surgical technique of choice (see Paidas, 1994) because it is associated with a lower risk of infection. If the abdomen cannot be closed immediately (if for example there is a large defect, bowel distension or oedema, or a small abdominal or chest cavity), the viscera can be enclosed within a silicone rubber ('Silastic') bag sutured around the edges of the abdominal defect and then returned to the abdomen over a few days ('staged procedure'). The abdomen is then closed at about a week. Other less common options for large defects include skin cover without fascial closure or over a Goretex patch, and non-operative closure by encouraging 'epithelialization' with daily application of 'Op-site' or antibiotics such as neomycin, bacitricin or sulfadiazine (see Langer, 1996).

The anaesthetic plan needs to consider the following:

a. The principles of anaesthesia for any neonate – e.g. differences in pharmacology and physiology; effects of prematurity; risks of hypothermia, hypoglycaemia, hypocalcaemia, and reversion to transitional circulation; the need for vitamin K prophylaxis etc.
b. The presence of additional congenital anomalies – e.g. congenital heart disease; Beckwith–Weidemann syndrome (Suan *et al.*, 1996).
c. The implications of the surgical condition itself – e.g. the risks of pulmonary aspiration of the bowel contents; a potentially large blood and fluid loss with gastroschisis; effects of an increase in intra-abdominal pressure on renal function, perfusion of the legs, ventilation.

Specific points of anaesthetic technique

General anaesthesia with muscle relaxation and positive pressure ventilation of the lungs is most commonly used, although subarachnoid anaesthesia has been described for repair of gastroschisis.

Large volumes of fluid are sequestered within the lumen of the bowel. Immediately before induction of anaesthesia the gastric tube should be aspirated to reduce the volume of stomach contents and the risk of pulmonary aspiration. The circulating volume should be reassessed (see above), and an additional 10–20 ml/kg of warmed albumin or a balanced salt solution given if indicated. The risk of pulmonary aspiration may be reduced by applying cricoid pressure as part of a rapid sequence induction. Cricoid pressure is effective in babies and, if applied correctly, should allow ventilation of the lungs without distending the stomach. It can, however, distort the anatomy or compress the trachea, making it difficult see the larynx at laryngoscopy or pass the tube into the trachea. If problems arise, cricoid pressure should be adjusted or released to allow intubation and oxygenation. The dose of induction agent should be reduced (e.g. thiopentone 3 mg/kg) because new-borns are more sensitive, but the dose of suxamethonium increased (2 mg/kg) to compensate for a larger volume of distribution.

During maintenance of anaesthesia nitrous oxide should not be used because it will distend the bowels and make it difficult to return them to the abdominal cavity. The choice of volatile agents and analgesic technique will depend on the likelihood of extubation at the end of surgery. Most babies are given muscle relaxants and their lungs electively ventilated for several days after repair of gastroschisis and moderate or large exomphalos. It is, therefore, unnecessary to use agents and drugs with rapid recovery characteristics. Maintenance with isoflurane or halothane (0.5–1.0 minimum alveolar concentration) in oxygen-enriched air and muscle paralysis with atracurium or vecuronium would be appropriate. You can provide analgesia with fentanyl. A minimum of 10 μg/kg is needed to prevent a cardiovascular response to surgery if no volatile agent is used. Some authors recommend doses of up to 100 μg/kg to reduce the stress response to surgery. This needs to be given over at least 30 minutes to reduce the risk of chest wall rigidity. The elimination of fentanyl is significantly prolonged by a rise in intra-abdominal pressure caused by a primary repair of gastroschisis. Extradural analgesia is probably less appropriate if the baby is ventilated after surgery, because infusions of morphine are commonly given to facilitate positive pressure ventilation.

Babies with a small exomphalos and no significant associated medical conditions may be extubated at the end of the repair. Maintenance with desflurane in oxygen and air and muscle relaxation with atracurium and regional analgesia using a lumbar-thoracic or caudo-thoracic epidural technique is probably the optimal technique for rapid recovery. Doses of bupivacaine should not exceed 2–2.5 mg/kg initially and 0.25 mg/kg per hour (either as a continuous infusion or repeat injection) post-operatively. Epidural bupivacaine should probably not be given for more than 36 hours in neonates because of concerns about the accumulation of local anaesthetic.

Blood and fluid losses can be large during repair of gastroschisis, and it is wise to insert a second intravenous (i.v.) cannula before surgery starts (size 22G minimum). One i.v. cannula can be used for maintenance fluids and drugs, and the other to replace blood and third space losses. Blood should be replaced with a balanced salt solution (3 ml for every ml of blood) or albumin (1 ml for every ml of blood). The acceptable blood loss is calculated by:

$$\frac{(\text{preoperative Hb} - \text{acceptable Hb})}{(\text{mean of preoperative and acceptable Hb})} \times \text{circulating blood volume}$$

Measuring blood loss accurately in small babies is difficult, and this should be used only as a guide. The acceptable haemoglobin is usually taken as 14 g/dl. Lower concentrations are associated with postoperative apnoea in premature babies. Fresh frozen plasma should be given only for a documented or anticipated coagulopathy (e.g. large blood loss in a septic baby). Third space losses should be replaced using a minimum of 10 ml/kg per hour of crystalloid (e.g. 0.9% saline) or colloid during surgery. Additional volumes will be needed postoperatively; the amounts should be judged according to the clinical condition of the baby. Gastroschisis is associated with hypoperistalsis and poor gastrointestinal absorption, and many surgeons insert a central venous line (e.g. a Hickmann line) for postoperative feeding. This line can be transduced intraoperatively; central venous pressure measurements may be useful in determining the type of closure (see below).

Most problems during primary closure are due to an excessive rise in intra-abdominal pressure (greater than 20 mmHg) causing a reduced cardiac output, hypotension and tachycardia; venacaval compression; decreased venous return; decreased aortic pressure and impaired perfusion of intra-abdominal organs; and impaired pulmonary ventilation. Some anaesthetists suggest using an infusion of dopamine 3–5 μg/kg per minute to maintain renal and gastrointestinal perfusion. If the baby deteriorates the surgeon may abandon a primary closure. The decision between primary closure and a staged repair is made on:

a. Clinical criteria – e.g. a diagnosis of abdomino-visceral disproportion; deterioration in ventilation (rise in end tidal CO_2, fall in oxygen saturation and pulmonary compliance); hypotension; dusky colour of the legs or abdomen; excessive tenseness of the abdominal wall etc.
b. Objective criteria – e.g. intragastric pressures greater than 20 mmHg or intravesical pressures; central venous pressure rise of 4 mmHg; end tidal CO_2 greater than 50mm Hg.

Intra-abdominal pressure may rise excessively after surgery, compromising the blood supply to intra-abdominal organs. Immediate postoperative complications include reduced pulmonary compliance and ventilatory failure; cardiovascular instability; bowel ischaemia and infarction; renal failure; sepsis; obstruction of the inferior vena cava; and impaired circulation to the legs. The resulting hypoxia and acidosis may reverse cardiac shunts.

Key learning points

- Abdominal wall defects are associated commonly with other significant congenital anomalies, of which congenital heart

disease and skeletal abnormalities have most significance for the anaesthetist.
- Treatment priorities are management of respiratory failure, fluid resuscitation, and the reduction of heat loss, further fluid losses and bowel distension.

Further reading

DYKES, E. H. (1996). Prenatal diagnosis and management of abdominal wall defects. *Sem. Ped. Surg.*, **5**, 90–94.

ENGSTROM, W., LINDHAM, S., SCHOFIELD, P. *et al.* (1988). Wiedemann–Beckwith syndrome. *Eur. J. Ped.*, **147**, 450–57.

LANGER, J. C. (1996). Gastroschisis and omphalocele. *Sem. Ped. Surg.*, **5**, 124–8.

PAIDAS, M. J., CROMBLEHOLME, T. M., ROBERTSON, F. M. *et al.* (1994). Prenatal diagnosis and management of the fetus with an abdominal wall defect. *Sem. Perinatol.*, **18**, 196–214.

SUAN, C., OJEDA, R., GARCIA-PERLA, R. O. *et al.* (1996). Anaestheia and the Beckwith–Wiedemann syndrome. *Paed. Anaesth.*, **6**, 231–3.

Case 7

A new-born baby is referred to the regional neonatal surgical unit with a provisional diagnosis of tracheo-oesophageal fistula.

Questions

1. Describe the structural abnormalities found in tracheo-oesophageal fistula (TOF) and oesophageal atresia (OA). How is the diagnosis usually made?
2. What are the important points in your assessment for anaesthesia? List the investigations required and discuss pre-operative preparation.
3. Discuss the factors affecting your anaesthetic technique and immediate postoperative care. What are the options for analgesia?
4. Describe the important postoperative complications.

28

Answers

1. There are six types of congenital oesophageal atresia. Most are associated with a fistula between the trachea and oesophagus (Spitz *et al.*, 1994):

   Isolated OA, either obliteration (type I) or atresia (type II) 7%
   OA with proximal TOF (type IIIa) 1%
   OA and distal TOF (type IIIb) 85%
   OA with proximal and distal TOF (type IIIc) 3%
   H-type (TOF without OA) (type IV) 4%

   The fistula, if present, lies on the posterior wall of the trachea, usually in the mid-trachea (59 per cent). Sometimes it arises distally (above the carina in 22 per cent, at the carina in 10 per cent, or from a bronchus in 1 per cent). Multiple fistulae may be present.

   OA or TOF is suggested pre-natally by the presence of maternal polyhydramnios or an absent or very small gastric fluid bubble and little intestinal fluid on ultrasound scan of the foetus. After birth, the diagnosis is suspected in a baby who drools excessively or coughs, splutters or becomes cyanosed whilst feeding (see Myers and Beasley, 1991). If the baby has OA it is impossible to pass a nasogastric tube and on X-ray it will be seen curled up in the upper pouch (if it is radio-opaque) with an air bubble in the stomach if there is an associated TOF. Contrast studies are not used because of the risk of soiling of the airway. Diagnosis of an H-type fistula is more difficult and is often delayed.

2. In the preoperative assessment and preparation of this baby, consider the following: the principles of management of any neonate for surgery; the presence of associated abnormalities; and the implications of the TOF or OA.

The assessment and preoperative management of any baby for surgery

Find out the baby's post-conceptional age; perinatal history (e.g. presence of foetal distress, birth hypoxia, respiratory distress syndrome etc.), type of delivery and any complications, and the weight.

Routine investigations and laboratory tests include: full blood count; urea and electrolytes; serum ionized calcium; blood glucose concentration and a cross match for blood. The haemoglobin (Hb) concentration is about 18.4 g/dl on day one and 17.0 g/dl on day seven in full-term babies. The Hb also depends on the amount transfused from, or lost to, the placenta at delivery. Blood glucose and calcium should be monitored. Hypoglycaemia occurs often in premature or growth-retarded babies, those who are seriously ill (e.g. birth asphyxia, hypothermia), or those born to mothers who are diabetic. A low ionized calcium can occur in severely ill babies or those born to diabetic mothers.

Sedative premedication is not required. If the baby has been born prematurely and extubation is planned at the end of surgery, caffeine 10 mg/kg may be given intravenously to reduce the risk of postoperative apnoea. It is important to ensure that the baby has been given vitamin K. Stores of vitamin K are low at birth, and bleeding can occur because of depletion of factors II, VII, IX, and X. Plasma concentrations of clotting factors are 30–60 per cent of adult values at birth, and do not achieve adult concentrations until 2–12 months, depending on the factor. Vitamin K partially reverses hypothrombinaemia within hours, and 0.5–1.0 mg is usually given intramuscularly immediately after birth to reduce the risk of haemorrhagic disease of the new-born.

Associated abnormalities

Babies with TOF or OA are often born prematurely. Associated congenital anomalies (usually cardiac or other gastrointestinal) are common, and are the usual cause of death.

Congenital cardiac disease: 19–49 per cent of babies with TOF or OA have cardiac abnormalities (Mee, 1991), of which half are major (e.g. tetralogy of Fallot, double outlet right ventricle or coarctation). A diagnosis on clinical grounds alone is difficult; surgeons suspect an abnormality in only 25 per cent and cardiologists in 40 per cent of cases with cardiac disease. All babies with TOF or OA should have an echocardiogram before surgery.

Concurrent syndromes: TOF or OA may be part of a concurrent syndrome e.g. VATER or VACTER (Vertebral, Anal, Cardiac, Tracheo-oesophageal, Renal) sequence in 13 per cent or CHARGE (Colobomata, Heart disease, choanal Atresia, growth and developmental Retardation, Genital hypoplasia, Ear abnormalities and deafness) syndrome in 16 per cent of cases. Retrognathia is common in CHARGE syndrome, and may cause problems with tracheal intubation.

Complex abnormalities of the airway: TOF with OA is associated with potentially fatal abnormalities, e.g. tracheal agenesis or stenosis, laryngeal atresia, pulmonary agenesis. Non-fatal abnormalities are common, and include ectopic right upper bronchus, trifurcated trachea and congenital bronchial stenosis.

Isolated OA and H-type fistulae are unassociated with other airway malformations.

The implications of TOF and OA

A baby with TOF or OA is at risk of aspiration. The risk is reduced by using continuous drainage from the upper oesophageal pouch (usually with a double lumen tube), nursing the baby in a head up position to reduce spill-over of gastric secretions, and not feeding. Check for pulmonary aspiration clinically and by examining the chest X-ray. Physiotherapy and appropriate antibiotics are occasionally required. The baby should be receiving maintenance fluids intravenously. Maintenance fluids are reduced in neonates during the first few days of life because of reduced glomerular filtration and adjustment in body compartments (in babies > 2.5 kg: day one – 60 ml/kg per day; day two – 90 ml/kg per day; day three – 110 ml/kg per day; day four – 130 ml/kg per day; day five – 150 ml/kg per day of water). Usually 5 or 10% glucose is infused, depending on the blood glucose concentration. Na, Cl and K are added after a few days.

Babies with TOF or OA are not operated on immediately. Clinical condition and pulmonary function should be optimized before surgery.

3. The anaesthetic plan should take account of the principles of anaesthesia for any neonate (i.e. adequately trained personnel, appropriate equipment, avoiding hypothermia etc.), and the specific considerations for TOF and OA.

Specific considerations

Leakage of gas through the fistula: In a baby with TOF there is a potential risk of preferential ventilation of the stomach through the fistula during positive pressure ventilation of the lungs, causing gastric distension, splinting of the diaphragm, pulmonary hypoventilation, impaired venous return and pulmonary aspiration. In clinical practice this is rarely a problem, and many anaesthetists induce anaesthesia with an intravenous agent (e.g. thiopentone) and a muscle relaxant. Others prefer to induce anaesthesia with a suitable volatile agent and intubate the trachea with the baby breathing spontaneously.

The fistula most commonly lies in the mid-trachea on the posterior wall, and ideally the tip of the bevel of the tracheal tube should be positioned along the posterior wall of the trachea occluding the fistula but allowing adequate ventilation of both lungs. The tip of the tube will lie low in the trachea with the potential for intubation of a main bronchus. Both lungs should be auscultated carefully to check for bilateral air entry after intubation and whenever the baby is repositioned.

If the fistula is very distal and associated with a large leak it may be possible to advance the tracheal tube into a main stem bronchus, preferably the left, and ventilate one lung until the surgeon has ligated the fistula.

The lungs should be ventilated with relatively low pressures to reduce air leak, but at an increased frequency to maintain normocapnia.

In the rare situation that leakage of gas into the stomach becomes a problem (e.g. low pulmonary compliance), the surgeon can make an urgent gastrostomy to relieve diaphragmatic splinting. However, this will not control the air leak and may not improve ventilation. Alternatively, the fistula can be occluded with a Fogarty catheter inserted from the trachea through a rigid bronchoscope or from the stomach and distal oesophagus. In an urgent situation, the surgeon can control the leak by opening the stomach and occluding the distal oesophagus with a finger.

Associated airway abnormalities: TOF with OA is associated with potentially serious abnormalities of the airway (see above). Some anaesthetists recommend premedication with atropine, pre-oxygenation, and intubation of the trachea with the baby awake, although this technique is more difficult and is associated with an increased incidence of hypoxia.

Nitrous oxide: Nitrous oxide will dilate the stomach and interfere with ventilation, and should not be used.

Patient position and surgical technique: Primary repair is the operation of choice, and the approach is extrapleural through a right lateral thoracotomy. The surgeon positions the baby on the left side. The anaesthetist must protect pressure points, confirm the position of the tracheal tube and ensure all monitoring is working. During surgical manipulation the baby's lungs should be ventilated by hand. The surgeon and anaesthetist need good communication. Oxygen desaturation occurs frequently because of pulmonary compression and ventilation–perfusion mismatch, and ventilation may become difficult or impossible because of compression or kinking of major airways. Occasionally surgeons mistakenly ligate or operate on structures other than the oesophagus or fistula. An attempt to ligate a right-sided aortic arch was identified when the reading from a pulse oximeter on a toe fell but that on the right hand did not.

The surgeon identifies the upper oesophageal pouch using a large suction catheter. Once identified, he or she will ask the anaesthetist to pass a smaller nasogastric tube into the stomach through the anastomosis, where it acts as a stent and allows early enteral feeding. This tube must be secured carefully, because it will remain in place for several days.

An H-type fistula is usually located in the cervical region, and is approached through an incision in the neck.

Intravenous access and fluid management: It is useful to have two intravenous cannulae (22G) in case one fails during surgery. One can be used to replace blood and third space losses (approximately 5 ml/kg per hour for a thoracotomy) and the other for infusion of maintenance fluids. Blood loss is usually minimal.

Monitoring: Standard monitoring as for any neonate should be used (i.e. electrocardiograph, non-invasive blood pressure, oxygen saturation, end-tidal carbon dioxide, core and skin temperatures etc.). A precordial stethoscope may help detect bronchial intubation or airway compression during surgical manipulation. Intra-arterial monitoring for blood pressure and blood gas, acid-base, electrolyte, glucose and haematology analyses is very helpful. Central venous access for perioperative monitoring and for postoperative fluid and nutrition is commonly used.

4. Postoperative ventilatory complications (e.g. apnoea and bradycardia, ventilatory arrest, aspiration, recurrent pneumonia) occur in about half the children. It can be difficult to identify the exact cause (tracheomalacia, gastro-oesophageal reflux or recurrent fistula) from clinical signs and symptoms.

   Tracheomalacia occurs in about one-quarter of babies with TOF. The cartilage of the trachea is deficient and does not give adequate support, and the width of the transverse muscle of the posterior tracheal wall is significantly increased (see Spitz and Phelan, 1991). The tracheal wall is abnormally weak and collapses easily. The diagnosis is suspected in a baby with a 'seal-like' cough, expiratory stridor, wheeze and airway obstruction worsening as the baby becomes upset. It may be associated with recurrent pneumonia. Symptoms start at 5–6 months of age, and usually resolve by 12 months as the trachea stiffens.

   In some babies the compliant trachea can become compressed between the aorta or inominate artery and the oesophagus, producing severe airway obstruction. The 'death attacks' or 'dying spells' often occur during or shortly after feeding in babies at 2–3 months of age, and are characterized by cyanosis, bradycardia and apnoea requiring resuscitation.

The diagnosis of significant tracheomalacia is made on bronchoscopy, during which the posterior wall is seen bulging into the tracheal lumen during expiration in babies breathing spontaneously. About one-third of babies with tracheomalacia will require aortopexy for symptomatic treatment of severe airways collapse. Aortopexy involves suspending the aortic arch from the posterior sternum at the sternal angle, pulling it away from the trachea.

Pulmonary aspiration can occur because of abnormal oesophageal peristalsis or gastro-oesophageal reflux.

Recurrent fistula occurs in 13 per cent of patients.

Other complications include anastomotic leak and stricture formation. Anastomotic leak occurs particularly after primary repair of atresia with a 'long gap' between the distal and proximal oesophagus. The risk is probably reduced if the baby is paralysed and its lungs mechanically ventilated after surgery. Stricture formation after repair of a 'long gap' is common, regardless of elective post-operative ventilation.

Key learning points

- Most tracheo-oesophageal fistulae are distal and are associated with oesophageal atresia.
- Common associated anomalies are cardiac and midline defects, and airway abnormalities.
- Anaesthetic management priorities include minimizing leakage of gas via the fistula.

Further reading

MEE, R. B. B. (1991). Congenital heart disease. In: *Oesophageal Atresia* (S. W. Beasley, N. A. Myers and A. W. Auldist, eds), Ch. 15, pp. 229–39. Chapman & Hall Medical.
MYERS, N. A. and BEASLEY, S. W. (1991). Diagnosis. In: *Oesophageal Atresia* (S. W. Beasley, N. A. Myers and A. W. Auldist, eds), Ch. 6, pp. 77–92. Chapman & Hall Medical.
SPITZ, L. and PHELAN, P. D. (1991). Tracheomalacia. In: *Oesophageal Atresia* (S. W. Beasley, N. A. Myers and A. W. Auldist, eds), Ch. 22, pp. 331–40. Chapman & Hall Medical.
SPITZ, L., KIELY, E. M., MORECROFT, J. A. *et al.* (1994). Oesophageal atresia: at-risk groups for the 1990s. *J. Ped. Surg.*, **29**, 723–5.

Case 8

A 12-year-old girl weighing 32 kg, presents for appendicectomy.
She has had abdominal pain for 3 days. The patient is fully alert, is
tachycardic with a heart rate of 140 beats per minute and a blood
pressure of 105/70, is dehydrated and in considerable pain. There
is concern about perforation of an appendix abscess and the
surgeon is keen to operate as soon as possible. The child is asthmatic and has been admitted to hospital on several occasions with
acute severe asthma. She takes regular salbutamol by inhaler,
salmeterol (a long-acting beta-adrenergic agent) 50 μg at night,
inhaled beclomethasone diproprionate 100 μg four times daily,
and sodium cromoglycate 10 mg four times daily.

Questions

1. What is asthma?
2. Which drugs are usually used in treatment?
3. What potential problems does it present to the anaesthetist?
4. Outline an appropriate perioperative management plan for
   this patient.

Answers

1. Asthma is a disease involving variation in intrathoracic airway
   obstruction, which occurs spontaneously or as a result of treatment. Measurements of airway function are difficult in children, and a working clinical definition of asthma is persistent
   or episodic wheeze, often accompanied by cough, when
   other likely causes have been excluded. About 10–15 per
   cent of school children in the UK suffer from asthma at any
   one time, and 20–25 per cent may have it at some time
   during childhood. The incidence of the disease is increasing.
   Episodes of wheeze are associated with bronchial smooth
   muscle constriction, inflammation and oedema of the bronchial wall, and mucus plugging of bronchioles. These changes
   occur in large and small airways, but peripheral airway
   obstruction seems to predominate in severe asthma. There
   are increased numbers of inflammatory cells, particularly
   eosinophils and mast cells, in the airways. Triggers for episodes
   of bronchospasm include infection, exposure to allergens,

exercise, cold, some drugs, and instrumentation of the airway during anaesthesia. Pulmonary compliance is decreased during bronchospasm, partly as a result of overinflation. Decreased compliance and airway obstruction increase the work of breathing and the accessory muscles may be recruited. Alveolar hyperinflation causes constriction of the intra-alveolar vessels with an increase in dead space fraction, and minute ventilation must increase to maintain normocapnia. Respiratory failure can occur if the work of breathing becomes excessive. Hypoxia is a consequence of impaired ventilation of alveoli that are obstructed and made atelectatic by bronchial obstruction.

2. Beta-adrenergic agonists act by increasing intracellular concentrations of cAMP in bronchiolar smooth muscle, which promotes relaxation. The phosphodiesterase inhibitors theophylline and aminophylline inhibit the enzyme phosphodiesterase and decrease the rate of breakdown of cAMP *in vitro*, but the concentrations required for inhibition of this enzyme are higher than those achieved during normal therapy. An alternative mechanism for their action is enhancement of the action of the non-adrenergic non-cholinergic inhibitory system in bronchial smooth muscle via adenosine receptors. Anticholinergics such as ipratropium bromide prevent the vagally mediated parasympathetic element, which can contribute to bronchoconstriction. Inhaled or systemic steroids inhibit the enzyme phospholipase A_2, which is involved in the production of mediators of bronchoconstriction such as leukotrienes and thromboxanes in inflammatory cells. They also suppress the release of inflammatory mediators from cells and enhance responsiveness to beta-adrenergic agonists, possibly by increasing the number of receptors on smooth muscle membranes. Inhaled steroids in children rarely cause adrenal suppression, oral candidiasis, laryngeal myopathy or growth impairment. When used systemically in severe asthma, steroids require 4–6 hours to exert an effect. Sodium cromoglycate acts as a mast cell stabilizer and reduces bronchial responsiveness. It is of no use in acute attacks, but has benefit as a regular prophylactic agent.

3. The main problem associated with severe asthma during anaesthesia and surgery is the risk of a severe episode of bronchospasm provoked by anaesthetic drugs or airway manipulations, which may result in severe hypoxia and the risk of pneumothorax during intermittent positive pressure ventilation.

4. The preoperative assessment should elicit a full drug history, including the use of oral steroids in the last 6 months, previous problems during anaesthesia, current drug therapy, visits to the GP, hospital admissions and any requirement for intensive care because of asthma. Examination can reveal indicators of severity, including obvious respiratory distress, persistent tachycardia after adequate fluids and analgesia have been given, pulsus paradoxus, widespread wheeze, and the inability to talk in complete sentences. The peak expiratory flow rate is of use, and can be compared with normal values if the child can cooperate – which is unlikely in this case. Pulse oximetry while breathing air is a valuable indicator of impaired gas exchange. Although this case is clearly urgent and a prolonged delay is unacceptable, some time should be spent improving the child's condition prior to surgery. The child should be adequately fluid resuscitated, and intravenous opioid analgesia given if required (morphine sulphate 50 μg/kg repeated as necessary until effective). A preoperative chest film will reveal any areas of infection that may be exacerbating the asthma, and provide a base-line for comparison if required in the postoperative period. A full blood count and measurement of plasma electrolytes should be performed. A nebulized bronchodilator such as salbutamol (2.5 mg/kg) should be administered. If there is no response to this, then intravenous aminophylline 5–7 mg/kg over 30 minutes may be given. If the child has received oral or systemic steroids within the previous 3 months, then hydrocortisone 1–2 mg/kg i.v. may be given prior to anaesthesia and repeated four times daily in the postoperative period.

Some of the normal subtleties and precautions employed when anaesthetizing for elective surgery in asthma are inappropriate in the emergency situation. Regional anaesthesia is inappropriate in this case, and endotracheal intubation with intermittent positive pressure ventilation is required. Once the child is adequately resuscitated and bronchospasm has improved, anaesthesia may be induced. Atropine may be given preoperatively to reduce the parasympathetic contribution to bronchospasm during the case. The child should be preoxygenated and anaesthesia induced with an intravenous agent. Some anaesthetists would prefer to avoid thiopentone in these circumstances because of concerns about histamine release, but it has been used uneventfully in asthma on many occasions. Similar concerns apply to suxamethonium for rapid sequence induction of anaesthesia, but for most people the risks of aspiration of gastric contents while the trachea is unprotected outweigh concerns about broncho-spasm induced by suxamethonium. Subsequent neuro-muscular blockade should be provided with an agent such as vecuronium, which does not release histamine. The trachea is intubated gently, but the cords should not be sprayed with lignocaine or lignocaine gel applied to the tube because of concerns about laryngeal incompetence in the postoperative period. Theoretically, the ventilator settings should have an inspiratory phase long enough to avoid high inflation pres-sures and a long expiratory phase to allow complete expiration. Anaesthesia is maintained with a volatile agent in oxygen and nitrous oxide or oxygen and air, and the F_IO_2 adjusted to main-tain an adequate S_pO_2. The volatile agent used is a matter of personal choice. All of the volatile agents are bronchodilators to some extent unless they are administered suddenly in high concentrations, when they can be very irritant to airways, and halothane is the easiest and smoothest to use. It has been shown to increase bronchial calibre, increase pulmonary compliance, reduce pulmonary resistance and improve gas exchange during asthma attacks. It may cause concern about dysrhythmias in patients who have recently been given sym-pathetic agonists or aminophylline, and some would prefer to use another agent. If analgesia has not already been given, it should be administered during anaesthesia. Morphine sulphate 0.1–0.2 mg/kg is commonly used. Concerns about histamine release lead some anaesthetists to avoid this and use pethidine or fentanyl, which cause less histamine release. Infiltration of the wound by the surgeon with 0.5% bupiva-caine is helpful. Some anaesthetists favour a high caudal block as a single injection, and a lumbar epidural may be con-sidered. If inflation pressures increase during surgery, then pneumothorax, endobronchial intubation, stimulation of the carina and blocking or kinking of the breathing system and tubing should be excluded before bronchospasm is treated. If this is thought to be the cause then increased volatile agent, nebulized salbutamol or intravenous aminophylline may be given, depending on which appears most appropriate in view of the child's previous responses. At the end of surgery anaes-thetic agents are discontinued, neuromuscular blockade is reversed and the child is allowed to wake before extubation. In an elective case extubation while the patient is still deeply anaesthetized may be preferred, but this is inappropriate if there is a risk of pulmonary aspiration of gastric contents.

Postoperative analgesia can be provided with an intravenous infusion of morphine sulphate (10–40 μg/kg per hour), or patient-controlled analgesia (PCA) may be used if the child is suitable, i.e. at least 8 years of age, has had adequate preoperative instruction in PCA, can use the trigger and understands the principles of demand analgesia and a lockout interval (bolus dose 20 μg/kg; lockout interval 5 minutes; with or without a background infusion of 4 μg/kg per hour). Again, although concerns are expressed about histamine release with morphine sulphate this is not a clinical problem in asthma, and changes of drugs and dosages and well-established ward routines to administer other opioids by infusion or PCA may be dangerous to the child. Non-steroidal anti-inflammatory drugs would usually be considered as contraindicated in this case, but a recent study of diclofenac in stable, treated asthmatic children showed no adverse effect on pulmonary function tests (Short *et al.*, 2000). Many children with asthma have in the past received NSAIDs such as ibuprofen with no adverse effects. Nebulized salbutamol 2.5 mg should be continued 2–4-hourly until the child is improved and can be managed with inhaled bronchodilators. If aminophylline is required, this is infused at 0.5–1 mg/kg per hour after the loading dose is given, with monitoring of the ECG and plasma levels assayed after 24 hours to determine dosage adjustments.

Key learning points

- The incidence of childhood asthma appears to be increasing.
- Preoperative assessment should include a detailed clinical history to gauge severity, precipitating factors and current medication.
- The usual priorities of safe induction of anaesthesia apply in the child with an intra-abdominal emergency and asthma.
- Most children with asthma tolerate analgesia with morphine well.
- A recent study of diclofenac in asthmatic children showed no deterioration in pulmonary function. However, caution is needed in severe cases, in the atopic child, in those with aspirin allergy and in those with asthma and nasal polyps.

Further reading

BRITISH MEDICAL ASSOCIATION AND THE ROYAL PHARMACEUTICAL SOCIETY OF GREAT BRITAIN (1998). *Drugs used in Treatment of the Respiratory System.* British National Formulary, Number 35.

GRANT, I. S. (1990). Intercurrent disease and anaesthesia. In: *Textbook of Anaesthesia* (A. R. Aitkenhead and G. Smith, eds), Ch. 41, pp. 645–76. Churchill Livingstone.

SHORT, J. A., BARR, C. A., PALMER, C. D. *et al.* (2000). Use of diclofenac in children with asthma. *Anaesthesia*, **55,** 334–7.

Case 9

A male child aged 12 weeks, weighing 3.1 kg, is listed for examination of the eyes under general anaesthesia followed by probable surgery to treat infantile glaucoma. The child was born at 28 weeks gestation by emergency LSCS for maternal pre-eclampsia. He was given surfactant at birth, ventilated in the SCBU for 6 weeks, suffered jaundice (which was treated with phototherapy), developed an episode of necrotizing enterocolitis (which was managed conservatively), received TPN and has been treated with oral steroids for bronchopulmonary dysplasia. He is nasogastrically fed, requires a low percentage of supplementary oxygen from nasal prongs to maintain an arterial oxygen saturation over 94 per cent, and receives diuretics and bronchodilators.

Questions

1. Is it reasonable for this child's anaesthesia and surgery to be deferred until he is 60 weeks post-conceptual age?
2. What are the problems with anaesthetizing this child for ophthalmic surgery?
3. How should the child be cared for in the perioperative period?

Answers

1. Infantile glaucoma may be caused by a primary congenital anatomical anomaly in the angle of the anterior chamber,

which interferes with the drainage of aqueous humour. A history of prematurity is common, and three-quarters of cases are bilateral. It may also be secondary to several causes, including uveitis, intraocular neoplasm, intraocular haemorrhage and trauma. If untreated, this condition leads to enlargement of the eye or buphthalmos because the immature sclera is unable to withstand an increased intraocular pressure. This is followed by oedema of the cornea and cupping of the optic nerve head, and rapid progression to irreversible loss of sight. Treatment is surgical and comprises trabeculectomy or goniotomy, which are intended to improve drainage of aqueous humour into the canal of Schlemm and reduce intraocular pressure. In view of these considerations, it is necessary to proceed.

2. This child is 40 weeks post-conceptual age and has several complications of prematurity, including bronchopulmonary dysplasia. There is a requirement to provide general anaesthesia with minimal effects on intraocular pressure caused either by drug administration or by manoeuvres such as endotracheal intubation during light anaesthesia, coughing, straining or vomiting. This is complicated by the fact that the child has several of the problems of prematurity that can make the provision of smooth anaesthesia difficult, and is at risk of postoperative apnoea from the effects of general anaesthesia. There is a high incidence of postoperative apnoea of between 30 and 40 per cent (range 0–82 per cent) in ex-premature infants undergoing general anaesthesia, particularly those of less than 44 weeks post-conceptual age, which is significantly higher than that seen in term infants. This susceptibility to postoperative apnoea is a result of immature respiratory control mechanisms, significant impairment of respiratory function in ex-premature infants until at least 1 year of age, airway obstruction, anaemia and the residual effects of anaesthetic agents persisting into the postoperative period. These residual effects of anaesthetic agents can reduce the chemoreceptor response to hypoxia, enhance paradoxical chest wall movement and contribute to depression of intercostal muscle activity. Recent evidence suggests that maintenance with the newer, more rapidly eliminated volatile agents is less likely to cause postoperative apnoea, especially if desflurane is used as the maintenance agent. The residual effects of muscle relaxants and opioids further depress respiratory drive and effort. A combined analysis of data taken from eight prospective studies in this population with a total of

255 cases undergoing general anaesthesia revealed that the main risk factors for postoperative apnoea were a low post-conceptual age, anaemia, and the occurrence of preoperative apnoeas. It was not possible to determine a post-conceptual age at which the risk of apnoea disappears, but no otherwise healthy child (without intercurrent disease) has suffered a postoperative apnoea after more than 60 weeks post-conceptual age. Once an apnoea has occurred, there is a risk of further apnoeas. Appropriate monitoring for an apnoea should continue for a minimum of 12 hours after operation or the last recorded apnoea.

3. The procedure must be performed in a hospital with the facilities to nurse the child in an appropriate manner to detect a postoperative apnoea should it occur, and with medical expertise to intubate the child and provide postoperative ventilation if required. Regional anaesthetic techniques are not suitable for ophthalmic surgery in ex-premature neonates, and a general anaesthetic is required. The laryngeal mask airway is unsuitable in this population and, in view of the child's respiratory problems, endotracheal intubation with neuromuscular blockade and intermittent positive pressure ventilation is indicated. This will allow the anaesthetist to prevent inadvertent movement or coughing, and to use a low inhaled concentration of volatile agent, remembering that the MAC value in preterm neonates decreases in proportion to the degree of prematurity. A suitable technique would be to fast the child for 4 hours preoperatively. Atropine or glycopyrrolate may be given by mouth 1 hour preoperatively. Given the problems of establishing venous access in this group of patients and the effects on intraocular pressure of a struggling child, an inhalational induction of anaesthesia is preferable, using halothane or sevoflurane. Once the child is asleep, a vein can be cannulated and neuromuscular relaxant administered. Endotracheal intubation may provoke coughing and straining if attempted under inhalational anaesthesia alone, and is best avoided. The use of a topical local anaesthetic solution such as amethocaine eye drops will provide early postoperative analgesia and avoid the need for opioid administration. At the end of surgery, neuromuscular blockade is reversed and the pharynx and nostrils are carefully suctioned. Some anaesthetists advocate giving lidocaine 1.5 mg/kg intravenously to depress laryngeal reflexes and increase the chances of extubating the child without coughing or laryngospasm. Caffeine 10 mg/kg intravenously may also be used to

reduce the incidence and severity of postoperative apnoea. Postoperatively the child can feed as normal, and post-operative analgesia is provided by paracetamol 15 mg/kg by mouth or nasogastric tube. The child should be nursed in a high dependency or intensive care area with an apnoea alarm to detect central apnoea and a pulse oximeter to detect hypoxia and bradycardia caused by an obstructive apnoea.

Key learning points

- Ex-preterm infants are at risk of perioperative apnoea up to 60 weeks post-conception.
- Postoperative monitoring in a high dependency or intensive care facility for a minimum of 12 hours is recommended.
- Measures to reduce postoperative apnoea in the ex-preterm infant include avoiding anaemia, and the use of caffeine and of modern volatile agents.

Further reading

BRETT, C. M., ZWASS, M. S. and FRANCE, N. K. (1994). Eyes, ears, nose, throat, and dental surgery. In: *Pediatric Anaesthesia* (G. A. Gregory, ed.), Ch. 21, pp. 657–97. Churchill Livingstone.

O'BRIEN, K., ROBINSON, D. N. and MORTON, N. S. (1998). Induction and emergence in infants less than 60 weeks post-conceptual age: a comparison of thiopentone, halothane, sevoflurane and desflurane. *Br. J. Anaesth.*, **80**, 456–9.

STEWARD, D. J. (1982). Preterm infants are more prone to complications following minor surgery than are term infants. *Anesthesiology*, **56**, 304–6.

Case 10

A 10-year-old boy weighing 24 kg, with a long history of ulcerative colitis, presents for an emergency colectomy after 5 days of conservative management of toxic megacolon. He presented with abdominal pain and fulminant colitis, and has been managed with intravenous fluids, parenteral nutrition, intravenous antibiotics and intravenous steroids. He has undergone numerous general anaesthetics for investigations concerned with his ulcerative colitis. On examination, he is lethargic, in pain, has dry mucous membranes and has not passed urine for

10 hours. His heart rate is 115 beats per minute, and blood pressure 105/55 mmHg. A full blood count is: Hb, 9.5 g/dl; WBC, 13.3×10^9/l; platelets 122×10^9/l. Electrolytes are: Na, 142 mmol/l; K, 3.3 mmol/l; Cl, 98 mmol/l; U, 8.7 mmol/l; creatinine, 90 μmol/l. A clotting screen is normal.

Questions

1. What is the pathophysiology involved in this case?
2. What problems does this child present for emergency anaesthesia?
3. How would you manage this child in the perioperative period?

Answers

1. Ulcerative colitis has an incidence of four to six per 100 000 children in the UK. It is an inflammatory disease of the large intestinal mucosa. Rectal involvement is seen in all cases, with pancolitis in over 60 per cent of cases. Macroscopically the mucosa appears granular and friable, and ulceration, haemorrhage, oedema and regenerating epithelium may be present with a bloody or mucopurulent exudate. Histological features are an acute and chronic inflammatory cell infiltrate in the lamina propria, distortion of crypt architecture, crypt abscesses and goblet cell depletion. Five to ten per cent of patients present with fulminating colitis associated with toxic megacolon. The aetiology of the disease is unknown. Psychological problems associated with chronic ill health, pain and diarrhoea, disturbance of schooling, chronic medication and frequent hospital attendance are common.

   Treatment of fulminating colitis involves nil by mouth, intravenous fluids, blood transfusion, albumin, intravenous steroids, broad spectrum antibiotics and, if the child is malnourished, parenteral nutrition. Surgery is indicated for failure to improve after 7–10 days, toxic megacolon, perforation, or significant colonic haemorrhage. Toxic megacolon occurs in less than 5 per cent of patients, and involves dilatation of the diseased colon with fever, tachycardia, hypokalaemia, hypoalbuminaemia and dehydration. A leucocytosis is present. Fever and tenderness may be masked by steroid treatment. There is a risk of colonic perforation, systemic sepsis and massive haemorrhage. In the emergency situation the most appropriate procedure is usually a colectomy with ileostomy, and surgery to restore continence is performed electively at a later date.

2. Likely problems in this case include:

   a. pyrexia, dehydration, toxaemia
   b. hypovolaemia
   c. anaemia
   d. hypokalaemia
   e. hypoproteinaemia
   f. intraoperative bleeding
   g. hypothermia
   h. risk of regurgitation and aspiration of gastric contents
   i. potential suppression of the hypothalamo–pituitary–adrenal axis
   j. postoperative pain.

In this child there will be oedema and swelling of the inflamed colon with a significant loss of intravascular fluid into the extracellular space, resulting in a deficiency of circulating volume.

A chronic anaemia is often present in inflammatory bowel disease because of poor dietary absorption and mucosal haemorrhage. Superimposed on this will be blood loss into the colon from areas of acute inflammation and mucosal damage in the colon.

Hypokalaemia is a consequence of gastrointestinal losses and inadequate intake of potassium.

Hypoproteinaemia and hypoalbuminaemia are consequences of chronic inflammation and poor dietary absorption with a severe acute illness imposed on this. They present a potential problem of unpredictable drug effects, since there may be less protein binding of drugs under these circumstances than normal.

Emergency colectomy is associated with significant blood loss as a large, swollen and inflamed colon is removed under difficult circumstances.

Heat loss during a prolonged procedure with a large abdominal wound and exposed surfaces may lead to hypothermia if precautions to prevent this are not taken.

As this is an emergency procedure in a stressed patient, despite the fact that he may be fasted there is a risk of reflux and pulmonary aspiration of gastric contents. Opioids and an ileus may contribute to this risk.

Postoperative pain in this case will be severe and require adequate treatment.

3. The child appears to be hypovolaemic and dehydrated, with anaemia. Although the blood pressure is maintained this may mislead, since hypotension is a late feature in children who are hypovolaemic and is an indicator that compensatory mechanisms are failing. Despite the fact that this is an emergency case, some time is required to resuscitate and prepare the child for surgery. Intravenous fluids consisting of repeated aliquots of 20 ml/kg of colloid or blood each given over 15 minutes should be administered, and the response assessed in terms of heart rate, blood pressure, JVP and urine output. Blood for transfusion should be cross-matched if this has not already been done. Analgesia may be given as morphine sulphate 50 μg/kg intravenously. The effect is assessed and the dose repeated after 10 minutes if required, until the child is comfortable.

A rapid sequence induction of anaesthesia is required. Once the child has been intubated and intermittent positive pressure ventilation commenced, then a large gauge secure peripheral intravenous cannula should be sited, a urinary catheter placed, a central venous line inserted (preferably in the right internal jugular vein) and possibly an intra-arterial cannula. A nasogastric tube to decompress and drain the stomach is required. Maintenance of anaesthesia may be with a volatile agent in air and oxygen, or intravenous agents with air and oxygen. An opioid by bolus or infusion is required – morphine sulphate 200 μg/kg (less if preoperative opioids have been administered), or fentanyl 2–5 μg/kg per hour.

During surgery, in addition to maintenance fluids, an allowance for insensible losses of about 10 ml/kg per hour is required and given as a balanced salt solution. Ongoing losses should be replaced as colloid or blood. Volume replacement should be titrated against heart rate, blood pressure, urine output, central venous pressure and the core–peripheral temperature difference. Measurement of haemoglobin during the case allows titration of red cell concentrate and plasma to reach a reasonable haemoglobin concentration. Large volumes of fluids may be required under these circumstances, and all fluids administered should be warmed to 37 °C. Prevention of hypothermia by the administration of warm fluids and the use of a heat and moisture exchanger, a warming circulating-water mattress and warmed-air insulating overblanket is required.

Postoperatively, loss of fluids to the abdomen will continue, and frequent assessments of volume status in terms of heart rate, blood pressure, urine output, CVP, peripheral perfusion and peripheral temperature are required. Additional boluses of fluid are likely to be required in addition to maintenance fluids to maintain circulating volume for 12–24 hours post-operatively. Given the requirement for invasive pressure monitoring and the potential for haemodynamic instability, the child would be best cared for in an intensive care or high dependency area. Many would electively ventilate such a case for a number of hours postoperatively.

Analgesia is probably best provided with an intravenous infusion of morphine sulphate (10–40 μg/kg per hour). Patient-controlled analgesia is an option in a child of this age if he is adequately prepared preoperatively and supervised postoperatively. However, in children who are very unwell the motivation and alertness required to use patient-controlled analgesia appropriately may be absent, and the technique often does not provide effective analgesia under these circumstances. Many anaesthetists would consider epidural analgesia contraindicated in a hypovolaemic child, and non-steroidal anti-inflammatory drugs should be avoided in patients who are hypovolaemic and at risk of renal impairment.

Key learning points

- An emergency colectomy in a child with ulcerative colitis is a high-risk procedure with potential for large fluid losses and compartment fluid shifts.

Further reading

JACKSON, W. D. and GRAND, R. J. (1994). Ulcerative colitis. In: *Principles and Practice of Pediatrics*, 2nd edn (F. A. Oski, C. D. DeAngelis, R. D. Feigin *et al.*, eds), Ch. 127, pp. 1863–9. J. B. Lippincott Company.

Case 11

A 6-year-old girl weighing 12 kg presented for Nissen fundoplication to treat severe gastro-oesophageal reflux. The child
had had severe cerebral palsy from birth and was severely
mentally handicapped. She was fed by nasogastric tube. Reflux
of gastric contents was copious, and made supplying adequate
calories in her feeds impossible and caring for her unpleasant
and difficult. She suffered recurrent chest infections thought to
be associated with pulmonary aspiration of gastric contents.
Haemoglobin concentration was 9.5 g/dl, white blood count
7.7×10^9/l and platelets 132×10^9/l. Chest X-ray revealed peri-
bronchial markings and basal atelectasis. Medical treatment of
her reflux had been unsuccessful.

Questions

1. What problems does this child present for perioperative
   management?
2. Describe an appropriate anaesthetic technique for this case.
3. What are the options for postoperative analgesia?

Answers

1. Severe gastro-oesophageal reflux, with or without a hiatus
   hernia, is common in children with severe cerebral palsy.
   Pulmonary aspiration may also occur because of poor co-
   ordination of the laryngeal muscles. These children tend to
   be malnourished because of the difficulties in feeding and
   obtaining adequate calories. Anaemia is likely because of oesophagitis, and chest infections are common. Venous access may
   be very difficult and epilepsy is not uncommon.
2. Preoperative preparation consists of optimizing the condition
   of the patient by correcting anaemia if present and providing
   preoperative chest physiotherapy and bronchodilators if
   required. Blood should be cross-matched. Premedication
   with antacids, metoclopramide and H_2 receptor blockers is
   often performed, but cannot be guaranteed to prevent reflux
   and pulmonary aspiration during anaesthesia. General anaesthesia with endotracheal intubation and intermittent positive
   pressure ventilation is usual. If there is a nasogastric tube,

this is aspirated prior to induction. In view of the risk of pulmonary aspiration of gastric contents, induction of anaesthesia should be by the intravenous route with cricoid pressure if venous access is available. If this is likely to be difficult and cause the child distress, then it is more humane to perform a gaseous induction and have an assistant obtain venous access when the child is asleep before administering a neuromuscular relaxant and intubating the trachea. A wide-bore nasogastric tube is then placed. Secure venous access is required for the case and for the postoperative period. If this is difficult, or postoperative parenteral nutrition is planned, then it may be appropriate to insert a central venous cannula after induction of anaesthesia to avoid prolonged and painful attempts at intravenous access by the junior staff on the surgical ward. Maintenance of anaesthesia with a volatile agent and intermittent positive pressure ventilation is required. It is common to omit nitrous oxide from the anaesthetic gases to prevent unnecessary distension of the bowel. Analgesia maybe provided by an intravenous opioid, a regional technique (most commonly an epidural), or a combination of the two. The child should be extubated awake to ensure that she is in control of her own airway.

3. These patients are high risk candidates for a prolonged and difficult postoperative course, and respiratory failure requiring postoperative ventilation may occur. The requirement for large doses of opioids in the postoperative period combined with an upper abdominal wound in a frail child with a bad chest is a poor combination, and there is significant postoperative morbidity and some mortality. Intravenous infusion of an opioid such as morphine sulphate 10–40 μg/kg per hour is a traditional method of providing postoperative analgesia. There is evidence that epidural analgesia is associated with fewer postoperative respiratory complications in this group and a reduced requirement for ventilation, and this procedure is a good indication for epidural analgesia if there is appropriate expertise and the hospital can provide suitable postoperative nursing facilities for a child with epidural analgesia. For upper abdominal surgery, the epidural catheter should be sited with its tip in the mid-thoracic region. An infusion of bupivacaine 0.125% to a maximum of 0.375 mg/kg per hour is suitable under these circumstances. This may be combined with an opioid such as fentanyl 2 μg/ml or morphine 1–4 μg/ml or an intravenous infusion of opioid (morphine sulphate 10–20 μg/kg per hour) administered simultaneously.

Non-steroidal analgesic drugs should be used if there are no contraindications. They reduce the requirements for opioids in the postoperative period and hence the likelihood of opioid-induced side effects, and improve the analgesia provided by epidural local anaesthetics. A low-dose benzodiazepine infusion may be useful in minimizing muscle spasm, e.g. midazolam 10–30 μg/kg per hour.

Key learning points

- Epidural analgesia is probably the best technique for children with cerebral palsy undergoing Nissen fundoplication.
- High dependency or intensive care is indicated for the immediate postoperative period.
- Chest physiotherapy is essential in the perioperative period.

Further reading

HOLL, J. W. (1994). Anesthesia for abdominal surgery. In: *Pediatric Anaesthesia* (G. A. Gregory, ed.), Ch. 18, pp. 549–70. Churchill Livingstone.
McNEELY, J. M. (1991). Comparison of epidural opioids and intravenous opioids in the postoperative management of pediatric antireflux surgery. *Anesthesiology*, **75**, A689.
MEIGNIER, M., SOURON, R. and LE NEEL, J. (1983). Postoperative dorsal epidural analgesia in the child with respiratory disabilities. *Anesthesiology*, **59**, 473–5.

Case 12

A 3-year-old girl with acute lymphocytic leukaemia (ALL) requires weekly bone marrow aspiration, lumbar puncture and intrathecal methotrexate injection according to her treatment protocol. She has developed a needle phobia and a general distrust of medical staff during her initial admission. Her parents are keen for her to have minimal fasting times and rapid recovery, and to be separated from them for the least time possible.

Questions

1. Discuss briefly the implications of the disease and its treatment regimen.

2. Is this child suitable for sedation or anaesthesia, and where should the procedure be performed?
3. How can the issue of her needle phobia be addressed?
4. Discuss some of the techniques available for use, mentioning the relative advantages and disadvantages of each.

Answers

1. Acute leukaemia is the most common paediatric malignancy with a peak incidence between 2 and 5 years of age. The national treatment protocols now used have markedly improved 5-year survival rates (greater than 60 per cent), but at the expense of the wider use of invasive procedures such as bone marrow aspiration, lumbar puncture and intrathecal injection of cytotoxic drugs. It is now no longer acceptable to hold down a screaming child in the ward treatment room to carry out such procedures. The most common complications arising from treatment and the disease itself are haemato-logical derangement and infection. Thus one may be presented with a child who requires a short sedative or anaesthetic, plus analgesia, at weekly intervals. The patient may be anaemic, thrombocytopenic and neutropenic, with a susceptibility to infection. In addition, the child may have become frightened of venepuncture and related procedures during the initial assessment, and careful subsequent management is required to regain both the patient's and parents' confidence.

2. Sedation and anaesthesia have been differentiated by the fact that verbal contact and airway reflexes are maintained during sedation but are lost during anaesthesia. Moreover, there is a continuous spectrum between the sedated child and the anaesthetized child, and it is difficult to predict the degree of sedation or anaesthesia that will ensue when the patient is given a particular agent. Despite the fact that a sedative regimen administered in a ward treatment room may be per-ceived as being more convenient and perhaps less traumatic for the child, it is perhaps safer to administer a short general anaesthetic in a controlled manner. This should be done by an anaesthetist using standard monitoring with a skilled assistant, usually in the operating theatre environment. If the list is properly organized and parents are allowed into the induction room and post-recovery area, minimal separation and fasting times can be ensured.

3. Venous access often rapidly becomes a problem in young children diagnosed as having acute leukaemia. It is now normal practice to insert an indwelling central venous line tunnelled through the skin. This is usually a double-lumen Hickman line or a subcutaneous reservoir system. The line can be used for drug administration and blood sampling, and its use has removed some of the stress of disease management. These lines should be inserted under general anaesthesia with image-intensifier control. Both laryngeal mask airways and endotracheal tubes have been used to secure the airway during these procedures. It is often more satisfactory to have intubated the child, in case the head and neck require repositioning or there is inadvertant large vessel puncture with consequent unexpected blood loss. Complications of using the lines are mainly infection (both localized and systemic), but also line displacement and blockage. It is important to use an aseptic technique when accessing the line, and also to flush the deadspace (volume depending on line size) with heparinized saline after use. Non-pharmacologic techniques such as play therapy, guided imagery and distraction are very helpful in this patient population.

4. A short-acting general anaesthetic for this child can be administered by a number of routes, using a single agent or a combined technique. Whatever technique is chosen, it is essential that fasting guidelines are adhered to and standard monitoring applied.

Intravenous agents

Propofol can be used as an infusion during total intravenous anaesthesia, or more simply given as i.v. increments during the short procedure. If a peripheral line is being used, it is important to add lignocaine (0.2 mg/kg) to the syringe to attenuate pain on injection. Propofol can be accurately titrated to the degree of stimulus, and allows for rapid recovery. It has the additional advantage of an anti-emetic property when used without nitrous oxide. An induction dose would be 4 mg/kg, followed by 1 mg/kg increments. There is often transient apnoea on induction, necessitating the presence of an anaesthetist and full airway management facilities. However, this is usually short-lived, and oxygen desaturations are rare.

Ketamine has both analgesic and sedative properties, making it a useful agent in this context. It also usually preserves airway reflexes and cardiovascular stability. However, it is not often used as the sole agent because it causes excessive salivation and also emergence excitation effects. Thus anticholinergics and a benzodiazepine such as midazolam are often added to the technique. The combination may mean the child takes longer to recover than when a single agent is used, and this may be less acceptable if early discharge and rapid return to normality is desired.

Midazolam as a short-acting benzodiazepine has a place in the provision of anxiolytic and sedative effects, but it will not result in anaesthesia or analgesia. Thus it can be used as a premedicant or in combination with ketamine as mentioned. The usual starting dose is 0.1 mg/kg. Methohexitone and etomidate have also been described as techniques for paediatric oncology procedure management, but appear to confer little advantage over existing newer agents.

Inhalational agents
If i.v. access is not pre-existing, it is often simpler to perform an inhalational induction on the suitably prepared child. With the introduction of sevoflurane, this can be well tolerated with rapid induction and emergence from a short procedure due to the low blood–gas solubility and minimal respiratory tract irritation of sevoflurane. Sevoflurane is now probably the agent of choice in this context, although the use of inhalational agents such as halothane has been commonplace until recently. This is despite the risk (albeit very low) of halothane hepatitis in the child, and it is perhaps now possible to avoid this risk. Sevoflurane can obviously be used as the maintenance agent if anaesthesia is induced intravenously.

Topical local anaesthesia
If the child does not have an indwelling central line, then topical local anaesthesia in the form of EMLA cream or Ametop gel must be used if peripheral access is to be sited. These agents also have a useful place in providing surface analgesia over the bone marrow or lumbar puncture site and decreasing the requirement for depth of anaesthesia during the procedure.

Key learning points

- A modern general anaesthetic best provides the requirements for such cases.

- Needle phobia can be minimized by the use of topical local anaesthesia, indwelling lines or reservoirs, inhalational anaesthesia, and techniques such as distraction and guided imagery.

Further reading

FERGUSON, S. and BALL, A. J. (1996). Sedation and sedative drugs in paediatrics. *Br. J. Hosp. Med.*, **55(10)**, 611–15.

HALL, S. C. and STEVENSON, G. W. (1990). Anesthetic considerations in the pediatric cancer patient. *Sem. Surg. Oncol.*, **6**, 148–55.

MARTIN, L. D., PASTERNAK, R. L. and PUDIMAT, M. A. (1992). Total intravenous anesthesia with propofol in pediatric patients outside the operating room. *Anesth. Analg.*, **74(4)**, 609.

Case 13

A 4-year-old boy presents for elective circumcision. He is known to be haemophiliac, and has an indwelling PortaCath central venous catheter for administration of factor VIII concentrate at home.

Questions

1. What is the aetiology of haemophilia, and what are its clinical features?
2. What are the likely perioperative problems in this child?
3. Suggest a plan of management for this child's anaesthesia and surgery.

Answers

1. Haemophilia A (or classical haemophilia) is one of the commonest hereditary bleeding disorders, with an incidence of 1/10 000–1/30 000. It is caused by a deficiency of factor VIII coagulation activity (VIIIc), and is inherited in an X-linked recessive manner. It is therefore almost always seen in boys. Its symptoms and clinical course depend on the level of VIIIc present in an individual patient. Levels of less than

2 per cent of normal are associated with severe disease, and patients present with spontaneous bruising, bleeding into soft tissues and haemarthroses. Mild disease with levels over 5 per cent of normal may only cause problems after surgery or major trauma. Prophylactic treatment with factor VIII concentrate given three times a week in severely affected children has been shown to reduce long-term joint damage. This requires secure central venous access for treatment at home.

2. The major perioperative concern is the risk of prolonged bleeding from the surgical site, and this must be prevented by the prophylactic administration of factor VIII concentrate before and after surgery. Further concerns are the problem of providing adequate analgesia when the techniques of caudal epidural blockade and penile nerve block are contraindicated because of the risk of haematoma, and non-steroidal anti-inflammatory drugs because of their effects on haemostasis. Depending on the child's origins and the origins of the blood products he has received in the past, he may be at risk of a transmitted disease such as hepatitis B, hepatitis C or HIV infection. Many countries now treat haemophiliac children with recombinant factor VIIIc, which is free of the risk of disease transmission, and in some areas a child of this age will never have been exposed to donor blood products.

3. Management of the haemophilia for elective surgery should be undertaken by the haematologist caring for the child. Although desmopressin is of use in moderate haemophilia to cover minor surgical procedures, this should only be used after preoperative testing of efficacy and dose response. Management will almost always involve the preoperative administration of factor VIIIc in sufficient amounts to raise levels to 80–100 per cent of normal. The dose required will depend on the child's weight, the level of factor VIII activity desired and the presence of factor VIII inhibitors. Administration will normally be repeated postoperatively to maintain levels of over 50 per cent normal until the child is considered not to be at risk of bleeding. Some recommend that a peripheral intravenous cannula should be placed after induction to avoid using the central line for anaesthetic drug administration. A laryngeal mask airway can be used for airway maintenance with spontaneous ventilation. Since regional techniques are contraindicated, the child should receive intravenous opioid in theatre while anaesthetized (morphine sulphate 0.1 mg/kg), and further increments of 0.05 mg/kg may be necessary in the recovery area until the child is pain free. Post-

operatively, analgesia may be provided by a combination of regular application of lignocaine gel 1 or 2% to the operative site, and paracetamol 15 mg/kg orally 4-hourly. Oral or intra-venous morphine may be used for severe pain. The child should be managed as an inpatient rather than a day case, and should stay for 24–36 hours postoperatively.

Key learning points

- Circumcision in a haemophiliac child will require full peri-operative work up and administration of factor VIIIc.
- Regional analgesia and NSAIDs are contraindicated.
- Topical local anaesthesia with lignocaine gel is non-invasive and extremely effective.

Further reading

KING, D. J. (1998). Disorders of the blood and reticuloendothelial system. In: *Forfar and Arneil's Textbook of Pediatrics*, 5th edn (A. G. M. Campbell and I. McIntosh, eds), Ch. 15, pp. 847–83. Churchill Livingstone.

NILSSON, I. M., BERNTORP, E., LJUNG, R. *et al.* (1994). Prophylactic treatment of severe hemophilia A and B can prevent joint disability. *Sem. Hematol.*, **31** (suppl. 2), 5–9.

Case 14

A 4-year-old girl is listed for closure of an atrial septal defect (ASD) using an occlusion device. The diagnosis of ASD had been made 6 months ago after her general practitioner heard a murmur whilst examining her for a chest infection. She is currently well.

Questions

1. Describe the different types of ASD and their clinical presentations.
2. Discuss your anaesthetic plan.
3. Discuss the possible perioperative complications.

Answers

1. ASDs account for 7 per cent of all types of congenital heart disease. An ASD can be classified into one of three anatomical types; a patent foramen ovale, or either an ostium primum or secundum defect (see Cooper and Goldstein, 1998).

Patent foramen ovale
The foramen ovale is functionally closed after birth by the left-sided septum primum opposing the septum secundum like a flap. The septa usually fuse sometime later, but this fails in about 50 per cent of children and the foramen ovale remains potentially patent. A patent foramen ovale can allow venous emboli to enter the systemic circulation (e.g. during a Valsalva manoeuvre), and is uncommonly associated with cerebral or coronary ischaemia. Children with high right-sided atrial pressures or a distended left atrium may re-open a potentially patent foramen and develop shunts.

Ostium primum defect
An ostium primum (or partial atrio-ventricular canal) defect results from failure of the septum primum to fuse with the endocardial cushions during embryological development. It is usually associated with mitral regurgitation because of a defect in the mitral valve. Severe pulmonary hypertension in an ostium primum defect often develops early, and may be symptomatic in infancy.

Ostium secundum defect
These account for 80 per cent of ASDs. The abnormality arises either because the septum primum partially resorbs during foetal development or the septum secundum is abnormally short.

An ASD produces a left-to-right shunt, with large increases in pulmonary blood flow. However, irreversible pulmonary vascular disease does not generally develop with a secundum ASD until adulthood, and tends to be asymptomatic in childhood. Occasional children have recurrent chest infections, and those with large shunts may complain of tiredness and shortness of breath.

On auscultation, a systolic murmur maximal to the left of the upper sternum can be heard, and fixed splitting of the second heart sound. With a moderate to large defect, increased flow through the tricuspid valve will produce a short mid-diastolic murmur to the left of the lower sternum. In an ostium primum defect there may be an additional systolic murmur at the apex caused by mitral regurgitation.

The electrocardiograph (ECG) in a child with a secundum ASD commonly shows partial right bundle branch block. If pulmonary hypertension is present, right ventricular hypertrophy may be seen on the ECG, and cardiomegaly or increased vascular markings on chest X-ray. Echocardiography may also show paradoxical septal wall motion, or confirm right ventricular hypertrophy. These features are associated with a shunt ratio (Q_p/Q_s) greater than 1.5. The ECG and chest X-ray features of right atrial and ventricular enlargement are more obvious with a primum defect.

The cardiologists can close a secundum ASD or a patent foramen ovale with an occlusion device if the defect has a diameter of less than 20 mm and is surrounded by a sufficient rim of tissue. The usual indications for closure are evidence of pulmonary hypertension or right ventricular hypertrophy as discussed above, or a right-to-left shunt. ASDs with small shunt fractions and no abnormalities of the ECG, chest X-ray or echocardiograph are closed increasingly commonly to prevent pulmonary vascular disease or atrial fibrillation developing in adulthood. The technique is inappropriate for a primum ASD or if the child has associated abnormalities requiring open heart surgery (see Allen *et al.*, 1998).

2. Children in some centres are managed for diagnostic and certain interventional catheters under sedation (e.g. oral premedication with chloral hydrate 75–100 mg/kg or midazolam 0.5 mg/kg and supplements of morphine or midazolam during the procedure) or light anaesthesia without protection of the airway (e.g. ketamine 0.25–0.5 mg/kg followed by 1 mg/kg per hour and midazolam 0.1–0.2 mg/kg followed by 100 μg/kg per hour). General anaesthesia with a laryngeal mask is possible, but intubation of the trachea and positive pressure ventilation of the lungs is usually required for ASD closure because the devices are guided more easily using transoesophageal echocardiography (TOE). TOE also reduces the doses of radiation and contrast. Inserting and manipulating the probe in lightly anaesthetized patients without airway protection is associated with excessive and unpredictable movement and airway obstruction.

   The majority of children suitable for closure of a secundum ASD with a device have good cardiac function, and, unless there are other indications, sedative premedication is not essential. Topical anaesthetics (e.g. Ametop or EMLA) applied one to one-and-a-half hours before the catheter will allow you to insert a cannula painlessly before induction of anaesthesia.

The choice of induction in children with reasonable cardiac function and a left-to-right shunt is not important; you can use either an inhalational or intravenous technique (e.g. sevoflurane or thiopentone 5–7 mg/kg and fentanyl 3–10 μg/kg or propofol 2.5–4 mg/kg). Theoretically, induction times are reduced with volatile agents but prolonged by intravenous agents in left-to-right shunts, but this is not important in practice. Reversal of the shunt is a likely risk only in children with marked pulmonary hypertension.

Ketamine 1–2 mg/kg is probably a more appropriate induction agent in children with poor cardiac function, pulmonary hypertension and right-to-left shunt.

Anaesthesia can be maintained with a volatile agent (e.g. isoflurane) and increments of fentanyl or with a propofol infusion technique with or without short-acting opioids such as alfentanil or remifentanil. The choice of muscle relaxant is not usually important, but pancuronium may be useful with reduced cardiac function. Antibiotic cover (e.g. cephalexin 30 mg/kg) is recommended for all interventional procedures. Heparin 50–100 units/kg is usually given to reduce the incidence of thrombosis or embolism, and a further 50 units/kg injected every 90 minutes (see Rheuban and Carpenter, 1998). Alternatively, the activated clotting time can be checked every 30 minutes and heparin given if it is less than 200 seconds.

Air must be scrupulously excluded from intravenous lines because of the potential for parodoxical embolus across the ASD. Some anaesthetists do not use nitrous oxide to reduce complications if air embolism does occur.

Maintenance fluids (e.g. glucose 5% and saline 0.45%) should be given at a rate according to accepted schemes. Intravenous lines and monitoring must be reliable, because the anaesthetist will have limited access to the child during the procedure.

Monitoring

Monitoring should be according to national recommendations. Some physiological variables can be affected in cyanotic heart disease (Purday, 1994):

a. Pulse oximetry overestimates a low haemoglobin oxygen saturation by about 5 per cent.

b. Capnography is particularly unreliable in the presence of shunts. The end-tidal CO_2 tension can be used as an indicator of gross arterial changes, but the arterial CO_2 must be measured formally to assess the difference between these values.

Discomfort at the site of insertion of the catheter can be treated with suppositories of paracetamol 30 mg/kg after induction of anaesthesia, and infiltration of local anaesthetic (e.g. bupivacaine 2 mg/kg).

After reversal of anaesthesia, these children should be transferred to a high-dependency unit for monitoring of physiological variables and observation of the catheter site for haemorrhage and peripheral perfusion. To prevent thrombi forming on the device before epithelialization, these children are given aspirin or warfarin each day for 3–6 months.

3. An occlusion device such as a double umbrella, button or double discs (see Allen *et al.*, 1998; Mendelsohn and Shim, 1998) is delivered over a guide wire passed through an introducer usually inserted into the femoral vein using a Seldinger technique. A femoral artery cannula is often sited to measure the blood pressure continuously. The *overall* incidence of important morbidity associated with cardiac catheterization (e.g. serious arrhythmias, cardiac perforation, significant haemorrhage) is 1.4 per cent, with an overall mortality rate of 0.9 per cent. Minor complications, such as non-life threatening arrhythmias or vascular injury, are more common (6.8 per cent). The rate of significant complications with ASD closure devices is about 5 per cent (Mendelsohn and Shim, 1998).

Contrast media
Conventional modern radiopaque agents are water-soluble preparations of organic iodide. They are viscous, but have a lower osmolarity than older agents and fewer side effects. They can aggregate red blood cells and are associated rarely with anaphylactoid reactions (see Rheuban and Carpenter, 1998). A low-grade fever 4–8 hours after the procedure is often attributed to the radiopaque dye (Mendelsohn and Shim, 1998). The dose of contrast should be limited to 5 ml/kg.

Arrhythmias
Arrhythmias, particularly atrial arrhythmias (e.g. supraventicular tachycardias, atrial flutter), and transient atrio-ventricular block

are common (Mendelsohn and Shim, 1998). They usually resolve spontaneously.

Vascular or cardiac trauma

Traumatic events such as perforation of the heart producing a pericardial effusion, laceration of valve leaflets or damage to major vessels and retroperitoneal haemorrhage are rare but can occur. Damage to vessels in the groin is more common with ASD closure because a relatively large venous line is needed to introduce the device. Transfusion of blood or colloid to treat haemorrhage is needed in 8 per cent of children. Femoral artery spasm or thrombosis are associated with a loss of peripheral pulses, a cool extremity, and a delay in capillary return. If signs persist for more than 2 hours, treatment with heparin (20 units/kg per hour) for 24–48 hours should be considered or, occasionally, thrombolytic agents (e.g. urokinase or streptokinase; see Rheuban and Carpenter, 1998).

Embolism of air, thrombus or the device

Pulmonary venous air embolus producing hypotension, arrhythmias, cyanosis and a decrease in the end-tidal carbon dioxide tension is a potential risk. If thrombi or air pass through the ASD they may enter the coronary circulation (producing ST segment elevation, hypotension, hypoxia and bradycardia) or cerebral circulation (producing strokes and recurrent seizures after the procedure) (see Mendelsohn and Shim, 1998). Thrombus can also form on the closure device, with the risks of cerebral, coronary or pulmonary embolus. The risk is reduced during the procedure by giving heparin and afterwards with aspirin or warfarin until the device is epithelialized (see Mendelsohn and Shim, 1998).

Occasionally the device may be lost from the introducer before it is secure within the ASD. Some devices are retrievable with a catheter, but others require surgical removal. Devices or their components may embolize late – e.g. a fractured arm of a double umbrella, or 'unbuttoning' of a button device (Allen *et al.*, 1998).

Residual shunt

Closure with a device sometimes fails (e.g. with defects greater than 20 mm in diameter or where the rim of tissue is insufficient). Residual shunting through the ASD occurs commonly after a device has been inserted, but leaks tend to resolve over time and are not usually haemodynamically important.

Knotting of catheters

Knots may make the catheter difficult or impossible to remove. There are special stylettes and retrieval devices for this situation.

Brachial plexus injury

Most cardiologists prefer the child's hands to be positioned behind the head with more than 90° of abduction at the shoulder to allow use of lateral cameras. Damage to the brachial plexus has been reported.

Key learning points

- Transcatheter closure is appropriate for most secundum ASDs.
- The anaesthetic technique is influenced by the use of trans-oesophageal echocardiography, which is most safely conducted in the intubated, ventilated child.
- The rate of significant complications is approximately 5 per cent.

Further reading

ALLEN, H. D., BEEKMAN, R. H., CARSON, A. *et al.* (1998). Pediatric cardiac catheterization: a statement for healthcare professionals. *Circulation*, **97**, 609–25.

COOPER, J. R. and GOLDSTEIN, M. T. (1998). Septal and endocardial cushion defects and double outlet right ventricle perioperative management. In: *Pediatric Cardiac Anaesthesia* (C. Lake, ed.), Ch. 14, pp. 285–302. Appleton & Lange.

MENDELSOHN, A. M. and SHIM, D. (1998). Inroads in transcatheter therapy for congenital heart disease. *J. Ped.*, **133**, 324–33.

PURDAY, J. P. (1994). Monitoring during paediatric cardiac anaesthesia. *Can. J. Anaesth.*, **41**, 818–44.

RHEUBAN, K. S. and CARPENTER, M. A. (1998). Diagnostic cardiac catheterization, angiography, and interventional catheterization. In: *Pediatric Cardiac Anaesthesia* (C. Lake, ed.), Ch. 6, pp. 69–84. Appleton & Lange.

Case 15

A 6-year-old boy has cut his fingers on a kitchen knife. He has sustained lacerations to the dorsal aspect of his left index and middle fingers.

Question

1. What are the different approaches to providing adequate analgesia for this boy?

Answers

1. There are a number of different ways of providing analgesia for this patient, and the decision will depend on important information about the child and also on the extent of the laceration in question.

   A full history should always be taken from the parents and the child, concentrating on essential points in the child's past medical history, previous anaesthetics (both general and local) and any adverse reactions that he may have had. Information regarding medication that he may be on and any history of allergies must be obtained. The fasting time of the patient must also be noted.

   If the laceration is superficial in nature and the surgeon involved is confident that there is no tendon or neurovascular injury, then the laceration may be cleaned and sutured if necessary in the Accident & Emergency department. The degree of distress the child is experiencing and the consent of the child and parents must be considered. The laceration can be anaesthetized by instilling topically a mixture of local anaesthetic and, if appropriate, a vasoconstrictor into the wound. Care is needed if the wound is on a digit, as the vasoconstrictor could be detrimental to perfusion of the territory of an end vessel. A dressing soaked in these agents may be applied to the wound. A recent study found that bupivacaine/noradrenaline was the most effective topical solution. It takes up to 20 minutes to provide effective analgesia, and further local infiltration of the wound with plain local anaesthetic solution from the anaesthetized surface outwards is easy and less upsetting for the child. Another possibility is to use topical creams or gels to anaesthetize small lacerations and their surrounding skin, although the manufacturers do not recommend this because systemic uptake from an open wound is more likely.

   If the cut requiring sutures involves an extremity, a local anaesthetic nerve block can be used. For example, if the injury involves a finger or toe, a digital or metacarpal nerve block will provide adequate analgesia. The area of skin where the nerve block will be performed can be anaesthetized using a topical preparation like EMLA cream or Ametop gel. Plain local anaesthetic solutions should be used.

Another alternative would be to perform the local anaesthetic infiltration or nerve block under the analgesic and sedative properties of nitrous oxide. The nitrous oxide can be provided in a pressurized cylinder as a 50:50 oxygen:nitrous oxide mixture (Entonox.). The child controls the delivery of the nitrous oxide via a specialized demand valve, and can use either a facemask or a mouthpiece in order to do this. This is an inhalational form of patient-controlled analgesia. As sedative techniques by definition require verbal contact to be maintained at all times during the procedure, this criterion is fulfilled. The level of sedation is completely controlled by the child. Maximum analgesia is obtained after approximately 2 minutes of inhaling Entonox. Due care must be taken if other sedative drugs have been administered, as nitrous oxide may potentiate their sedative effects. Nausea and vomiting can also be a problem with using nitrous oxide as the sole agent. Children do not require to be fasted if nitrous oxide is the only agent being used; however, if there is concomitant administration of other sedative drugs the child must be appropriately fasted as for a general anaesthetic. Nitrous oxide can also be delivered by a continuous-flow machine that can give up to 70 per cent nitrous oxide in oxygen (e.g. Quantiflex apparatus), and this can be highly effective.

There are certain groups of children who are not suitable candidates for nitrous oxide due to its diffusable nature. This means that closed air spaces within the body are at risk of expansion as nitrous oxide diffuses into the space faster than nitrogen is able to diffuse out. As a result, Entonox is contraindicated in children with bowel obstruction, pneumothorax or head injuries, especially if there is a risk of intracranial air. Those children with abnormal airways or congenital heart disease and those unable to cooperate or understand the technique (i.e. those less than 3 years of age or those with developmental delay) should not use Entonox for sedation.

Sedation using other drugs, such as short-acting benzodiazepines or opiates, may be used by those appropriately trained. As with all sedative techniques, appropriate monitoring is mandatory as well as proper patient selection and preparation. Adequate record keeping must be undertaken, and this also is true for techniques using Entonox. If sedative techniques are not appropriate, then a general anaesthetic may be required.

With all the techniques mentioned above, appropriate adjuvant analgesia should be administered in the form of regular paracetamol with or without non-steroidal anti-inflammatory drugs.

Key learning points

- Children with lacerations need to be carefully selected for attempts at repair in the accident and emergency department.
- Local anaesthetic techniques alone may suffice.
- Nitrous oxide is very useful in school-age children.

Further reading

MORTON, N. S. (ed.) (1998). *Acute Pain Management: A Practical Guide*. W. B. Saunders.
ROYAL COLLEGE OF PAEDIATRICS AND CHILD HEALTH (1997). *Prevention and Control of Pain in Children*. BMJ Publishing Group.

Case 16

A 9-year-old boy weighing 23 kg presents for elective laparoscopic fundoplication. He has severe gastro-oesophageal reflux, which is known to be causing oesophagitis, but his parents have persistently declined open fundoplication because of concerns about the risks of major surgery and about postoperative pain. He has undergone numerous upper gastrointestinal endoscopies under general anaesthesia, and is otherwise well.

Questions

1. What are the potential advantages of a laparoscopic compared with an open fundoplication?

2. What are the potential problems of laparoscopic surgery in a child?
3. Describe an appropriate anaesthetic technique for this case.

Answers

1. Fundoplication is most commonly required in children with severe cerebral palsy, a group where it has been shown to improve respiratory symptoms associated with gastro-oesophageal reflux. The open operation is a major upper abdominal procedure associated with considerable morbidity and some mortality. A laparoscopic procedure is intended to minimize these problems. The major advantages are minimal postoperative pain, no requirement for an intravenous opioid infusion or epidural analgesia postoperatively, and a reduced hospital stay.

2. Laparoscopic procedures are becoming more common in children, and the potential problems of laparoscopic surgery are similar to those in adults. Potential cardiovascular problems include a reduction in cardiac output because of increased intra-abdominal pressure from the pneumoperitoneum and compression of the vena cava. This fall may be manifest as hypotension and tachycardia or a metabolic acidosis in small children, even if an adequate blood pressure is maintained. If a head up tilt is used, this will accentuate these effects. Blood pressure is usually maintained by an increase in systemic vascular resistance associated with compression of the aorta. Hypotension occasionally occurs if a head up tilt is assumed, but responds to volume administration and atropine if associated with a bradycardia. These effects can be reduced by limiting the insufflation pressure to 10–12 cm H_2O. Hypertension and tachycardia may be seen during stimulating parts of the hiatal dissection if anaesthesia is inadequate, despite the fact that surgery is laparoscopic.

   Respiratory problems include a further fall in FRC in addition to that induced by anaesthesia. This is caused by diaphragmatic elevation, a reduction in chest wall dimensions, a reduction in muscle tone, and changes in intrathoracic blood volume. If the FRC falls below closing volume, there is an increased intrapulmonary shunt. There is a fall in arterial oxygen tension, but if supplementary oxygen is used this occurs on the flat portion of the oxygen–haemoglobin dissociation curve and the arterial oxygen saturation is not affected. There is a reduced pulmonary compliance secondary to carbon dioxide insufflation, and a need for increased inflation pressures to maintain normocapnia. Endobronchial intubation or carinal stimulation may occur as the diaphragm is displaced cephalad by the pneumoperitoneum. These changes are probably accentuated if the patient is placed in the head down position. There tends to be an increase in peak inspiratory pressure if pressure-limited ventilation is not used, and a progressive increase in end-tidal carbon dioxide if minute ventilation is not increased. This rise in end-tidal carbon dioxide is a consequence of the absorption of insufflated carbon dioxide and increased alveolar dead space. The accuracy of end-tidal carbon dioxide measurement as an indicator of arterial carbon dioxide tension may decrease during laparoscopy if there is an increase in the arterial–end-tidal carbon dioxide concentration difference. This may occur because of a reduced cardiac output, hypovolaemia, or increased respiratory dead space. Occasionally pneumothorax and pneumomediastinum have been reported in adults under-going laparoscopic surgical procedures, especially if the insufflation pressure is not limited to a low value.

3. Premedication is optional, and depends on the state of the child and the anaesthetist's preference. Some anaesthetists use antacid and/or prokinetic prophylaxis. Induction may be by a rapid sequence induction, or a gaseous or intravenous technique incorporating cricoid pressure is often used. An intravenous cannula is placed and a neuromuscular relaxant administered before the trachea is intubated, the presence of a leak checked and intermittent positive pressure ventilation commenced. A large-gauge (22–26 FG) orogastric tube or oesophageal bougie is placed to deflate the stomach and pro-vide a stent in the oesophagus for the surgeon to wrap the fundus around and prevent the formation of too tight a wrap. Maintenance intravenous fluids are required and, in view of the length of the procedure and the inconvenience of unexpected patient movement, an infusion of neuromuscular relaxant such as vecuronium 0.1 mg/kg per hour is useful. Anaesthesia is maintained with a volatile agent in oxygen and air. Alternatively an infusion of an intravenous agent such propofol may be given, using either a manual schedule or a computer-controlled infusion. The bowel distension caused by nitrous oxide hampers the surgical procedure, and it is therefore usually not used. Analgesia in the form of a single bolus of opioid (morphine sulphate 0.1–0.2 mg/kg

or codeine phosphate 1–2 mg/kg i.m.) or an infusion of fentanyl at 2–5 μg/kg per hour is given during the procedure. In the absence of contraindications, a non-steroidal anti-inflammatory drug should also be given. An effective anti-emetic such as ondansetron (0.1 mg/kg; maximum dose 4 mg) should be given to minimize the chances of postoperative vomiting. The procedure is performed in the lithotomy position with a degree of head up tilt. The insertion sites for the camera and surgical instruments are infiltrated prior to surgery by the surgeon with bupivacaine and adrenaline to minimize bleeding and provide postoperative analgesia. The large-bore orogastric tube is changed for a smaller, more comfortable nasogastric tube at the end of the procedure. Postoperatively, intravenous fluids are administered overnight and drinking commences on the first postoperative day. Analgesia is provided by a combination of paracetamol 15 mg/kg 4-hourly, a non-steroidal anti-inflammatory drug (diclofenac sodium 1 mg/kg 8-hourly) and an opioid (oramorph 0.3 mg/kg 4-hourly) given by the nasogastric tube. Occasionally a systemic opioid (morphine sulphate 50–100 μg i.v.) is required. Shoulder pain may occur as well as abdominal pain. An anti-emetic should be prescribed and administered regularly (ondansetron 0.1 mg/kg i.v., maximum dose 4 mg).

Key learning points

- Laparoscopic fundoplication causes minimal postoperative pain, no requirement for an intravenous opioid infusion or epidural analgesia postoperatively and a reduced hospital stay.
- Similar complications of laparoscopy are seen in children to those seen in adults.

Further reading

MANNER, T., AANTAA, R. and ALANEN, M. (1998). Lung compliance during laparoscopic surgery in paediatric patients. *Paed. Anaesth.*, **8,** 25–9.

ROWNEY, D. A. and ALDRIDGE, L. M. (2000). Laparoscopic fundoplication in children: anaesthetic experience of 51 cases. *Paed. Anaesth.*, **10,** 291–6.

SFEZ, M., GUERARD, A. and DESRUELLE, P. (1995). Cardiorespiratory changes during laparoscopic fundoplication in children. *Paed. Anaesth.*, **5,** 89–95.

Case 17

A 6-year-old girl weighing 25 kg is admitted to the intensive care unit. She is in a profound state of circulatory collapse. Vital signs show a tachycardia of 190/min and hypotension with a systolic BP of 50 mmHg. She has a palpable liver edge of 6 cm, and is noted to be cyanosed and tachypnoeic with a respiratory rate of 42 breaths per minute.

The patient requires full resuscitative intervention with intubation, ventilation, invasive monitoring and inotropic support. Blood results show a coagulopathy with a PT of 64 s and an APTT of 140 s; the liver function tests are also noted to be deranged. Renal function is impaired, with a urea of 23 mmol/l and a creatinine level of 220 mmol/l; CXR shows fulminant pulmonary oedema with evidence of cardiomegaly. An echocardiograph is requested and shows evidence of a dilated cardiomyopathy.

Despite escalating inotropic requirements the girl remains haemodynamically unstable. The regional transplant unit is contacted and notified of her condition. They are willing to place her name on the urgent transplant list, but are unsure as to when a heart of appropriate size will become available.

Question

1. What treatment options are available to act as a bridge to transplantation? Give a brief description of the different types and how they function.

Answers

1. There are two main treatment modalities that can be used for continuing circulatory support and can act as a bridge to heart transplantation; they are ECMO (extracorporeal membrane oxygenation) and ventricular assist devices (VADs).

    ECMO has its origins in the 1970s, when prolonged periods of full cardiopulmonary bypass were tried in adult patients suffering from severe cardiorespiratory failure. The technique has developed largely in the neonatal and paediatric population for the treatment of acute respiratory failure, and latterly as a means of cardiac support.

In venoarterial ECMO the venous drainage cannula is placed in the right atrium via the right internal jugular vein, and the cannula for reperfusion is placed in the right common carotid artery at its junction with the right innominate artery. Other vessels can be used – for example the femoral vein and artery – or direct chest cannulation can be obtained via a median sternotomy.

The venoarterial ECMO circuit is very similar to cardiopulmonary bypass. Blood is drained by gravity into a 'bladder'. The bladder has an approximate volume of 30–50 ml, and has a number of important functions:

a. It regulates flow through the circuit – i.e. if there is irregular flow and the venous return decreases, the bladder collapses and a servoregulator shuts down the pump.
b. Any air that has gained access to the venous side of the circuit is trapped in the bladder, therefore preventing systemic embolization.
c. It acts as the main site for blood sampling and drug administration.

From the bladder, blood is then pumped via an occlusive non-pulsatile pump to a membrane oxygenator through which sweep gas flows in order to regulate oxygen and carbon dioxide levels. A countercurrent heat exchanger is then used to warm the blood prior to it returning to the ascending aorta.

The circuit volume is approximately 500–650 ml. A number of processes must occur prior to starting an ECMO run. The circuit is first flushed with carbon dioxide; this is then followed by a crystalloid prime and then a further prime with either whole blood or concentrated red cells and albumin. The fluid is then circulated in order to stabilize the oxygen, carbon dioxide and pH, and once this is done heparin is added. The flows are initially started at 50 ml/min and gradually increased to 150–200 ml/min. While on ECMO, ventilation is reduced to 'rest' settings – i.e. F_IO_2 0.3 and a respiratory rate of 10–15/min, peak inspiratory pressures of 20 cm H_2O and PEEP levels of 5 cm H_2O.

The potential complications of ECMO are varied: 5–15 per cent of patients develop intracranial haemorrhage and approximately 15 per cent develop seizure activity. Cardiovascular instability and dysrhythmias can occur, as well as evidence of renal impairment; the renal dysfunction is usually as a result of the patient's condition prior to starting ECMO. Consumptive coagulopathy, along with haemorrhage and haemolysis, are well recognized complications of this supportive technique.

Ventricular assist devices (VADs) differ from ECMO circuits as they only support the circulation, and therefore an oxygenator is not part of the circuit design. These devices are only useful in children who have ventricular dysfunction and require single organ support. They work by controlling both the left atrial filling pressure and the left ventricular pressure. The VAD can control and reduce the left ventricular pressure and, by doing this, enhance left ventricular function and aid recovery if possible.

There are two main designs of VADs; pulsatile and non-pulsatile blood pumps. The inflow cannula's placement depends on the reason for using the VAD. If ventricular function is anticipated to improve, the cannula is placed in the left atrium; if, however, the VAD is being used as a bridge to transplantation, its placement is less important and it can be positioned directly in the left ventricle.

Pulsatile VADs act as blood sacs, which can be emptied either pneumatically or by using an electric motor to activate a pusher plate (Novacor™ Inc. Oakland, CA). The blood is directed into the arterial tree either by prosthetic valves (Pierce-Donachy pump™, Thoratec Labs and Abiomed, Inc. Danvers, MA) or by porcine xenograft heart valves (Heart Mate™, Thermo Cardiosystems Inc.).

Non-pulsatile pumps use a centrifuge system (Bio-medicus™, Eden Prairie, MN) where the blood is entrained by the centrifugal force generated by spinning blades or cones. As with ECMO, anticoagulation is required with pulsatile and non-pulsatile pumps, but full heparinization is not necessary. An implantable impeller device within the aorta is also under development.

As with ECMO, a number of complications can arise when VADs are used. These include right ventricular dysfunction, infection, the risks of anticoagulation and concomitant haemorrhage, as well as clot formation if anticoagulation is inadequate. Patients with probe-patent foramen ovale are at risk of shunting if the left atrial pressure is reduced below that of the right. An echocardiograph should be performed in order to exclude this condition. Finally, a diastolic vacuum can be created prior to chest closure which results in air entering the circulation; air can also be entrained via suture lines and central venous catheters.

Key learning points

- Perioperative extracorporeal support is becoming more common in patients undergoing surgery for congenital heart defects.
- Circulatory support can be provided by VAD and venoarterial ECMO.

Further reading

GOLDSTEIN, D. J., OZ, M. C. and ROSE, E. A. (1998). Medical progress: implantable left ventricular assist devices. *N. Engl. J. Med.*, **339(21)**, 1522–33.

LAKE, C. (ed.) (1998). *Pediatric Cardiac Anaesthesia*, 3rd edn. Appleton & Lange.

LEVY, F. H., O'ROURKE, P. P. and CRONE, R. K. (1992). Extracorporeal membrane oxygenation. *Anaesth. Analg.*, **75(6)**, 1053–62.

SCHERR, K., JENSEN, L. and KOSHAL, A. (1999). Mechanical circulatory support as a bridge to cardiac transplantation: towards the 21st century. *Am. J. Crit. Care*, **8(5)**, 324–37.

WARNECKE, H., BERDJIS, F., HENNIG, E. *et al.* (1991). Mechanical left ventricular support as a bridge to cardiac transplantation in childhood. *Eur. J. Cardiothor. Surg.*, **5(6)**, 330–33.

Case 18

A 10-year-old boy is admitted as an emergency with suspected appendicitis. He has been feeling unwell for 3 days, and has vomited twice. He has no other past medical history and is on no medication. He has not had an anaesthetic before. On examination, he appears flushed and has a temperature of 38 °C. He weighs 35 kg and is receiving Ringer's lactate solution intravenously.

You are asked to anaesthetize him for an appendicectomy, and plan a rapid sequence induction technique using thiopentone (5 mg/kg) and suxamethonium (1 mg/kg). After administration of the suxamethonium, you notice that his jaw is stiff to open. You manage to intubate with some difficulty, administer fentanyl (50 μg), and the surgeon is anxious to proceed with the operation.

Questions

1. What concerns do you have after experiencing difficulty in opening the mouth?
2. What is your choice of anaesthetic management in this situation?
3. Should this boy undergo muscle testing for susceptibility to malignant hyperpyrexia?

Answers

1. Jaw stiffness or masseter muscle rigidity (MMR) should always alert the anaesthetist to the possibility of malignant hyperpyrexia (MH) developing. MMR after suxamethonium has an incidence of between 1:100 and 1:400 in children. It has been defined as 'incomplete relaxation of the jaw muscles interfering with intubation after suxamethonium administration'. This assumes that the suxamethonium has been given in adequate dose (1–2 mg/kg; 3 mg/kg in an infant) and sufficient time has been allowed for it to provide muscle relaxation (60 s). It is most likely to occur if halothane is then subsequently administered as the volatile agent.

   MMR is a subjective clinical diagnosis, which probably manifests to different degrees in different patients. This explains why there is variation in the reliability of MMR to predict whether a patient will then progress to full-blown malignant hyperpyrexia.

   In paediatric studies, the association between MMR and MH has been quoted as being around 50–65 per cent. However, it is now recognized that increased masseter muscle tone is seen to some extent in almost all patients after being given suxamethonium, and this can make the decision on whether to assume MH susceptibility (and treat as such) a difficult one.

   MMR might also be seen in a previously undiagnosed myopathy, which will result in additional anaesthetic risks such as arrhythmias due to hyperkalaemia.

2. The choice of anaesthetic management must take into account the urgency of the surgery, as well as the possibility that the boy may go on to develop signs of MH. As the nature of MH susceptibility is unpredictable, it is considered inappropriate to continue 'MH triggering' anaesthetic agents after evidence of MMR on induction. If this were an elective case, it would be advisable to discontinue the anaesthetic and observe for

any evidence of MH developing (e.g. generalized rigidity, temperature increase, acidosis and increased CO_2 production). However, as the appendicectomy cannot be postponed, the anaesthesia should be continued with 'non-triggering' agents such as propofol using a total intravenous anaesthetic technique (TIVA) and oxygen and nitrous oxide. The anaesthetic breathing circuit must be changed, and all vaporizers removed from the anaesthetic machine. If further muscle relaxation is required, this can be provided with a non-depolarizing, short-acting agent – although, as mentioned, it should be borne in mind this boy may suffer from a myopathy. Full and vigilant monitoring for signs of MH should be in place, including core temperature and arterial blood gases. It is important to have dantrolene available and ready to be administered in an initial dose of 1 mg/kg. Mechanisms for immediate cooling of the patient should also be made ready. If the boy does not appear to show any signs of MH, he should still be monitored postoperatively on a high-dependency unit for 24 hours. If MH is considered at all likely, then the standard MH protocol is followed.

3. As the consequences of a full-blown MH reaction are so catastrophic and MMR has such strong links with MH, all suspected cases must be investigated regardless of age. *In vitro* testing of muscle contracture to halothane and caffeine is considered standard. This test achieves high sensitivity and acceptable specificity when performed in the laboratory of a specialist centre. Using 'MH trigger-free' anaesthesia or a regional technique, the boy should have a strip of vastus muscle excised. Pieces of this are then exposed to both halothane and caffeine and the tension that is generated by the muscle strips measured. If he is MH susceptible, greater tensions will occur at lower concentrations of testing agents. If this is the case, the boy's family should be tested in the same way, starting with first-degree relatives. The patient, his family and his GP must be fully informed of the test results and possible diagnosis.

Key learning points

- Masseter spasm should prompt further invesigation.
- If anaesthesia has to proceed, adopt a trigger-free technique.
- The child should be observed in a high-dependency or intensive care unit for at least 24 hours.

Further reading

HOPKINS, P. M. (1999). Malignant hyperthermia. CME core topic. *Royal College of Anaesthetists Newsletter*, **46,** 99–103.

ROSENBERG, H. (1987). Trismus is not trivial (editorial). *Anesthesiology*, **67,** 453–5.

ROSENBERG, H. and SHUTACK, J. G. (1996). Variants of malignant hyperpyrexia. Special problems for the paediatric anaesthesiologist. *Paed. Anaesth.*, **6,** 87–93.

O'FLYNN, R. P., SHUTACK, J. G, ROSENBERG, H. and FLETCHER, J. E. (1994). Masseter muscle rigidity and malignant hyperthermia susceptibility in pediatric patients: an update on management and diagnosis. *Anesthesiology*, 80, 1228–33.

Case 19

As a locum anaesthetist in a hospital that undertakes low-risk births but does not provide a dedicated obstetric anaesthetic service or on site paediatric facilities, you are asked to attend the labour of a woman where meconium staining of the amniotic fluid has been seen by the midwife and delivery is imminent. The child is 41 weeks gestation to a 1 + 1 mother after an uneventful pregnancy. The initial Apgar score is 6 and at 5 minutes it is 4.

Questions

1. What is the Apgar score?
2. What is meconium aspiration syndrome?
3. Describe the principles of neonatal resuscitation in the labour ward.

Answers

1. The Apgar score is an objective method of diagnosing birth asphyxia. Five variables that are easily elicited are each given scores from 0–2 at 1 minute and 5 minutes after birth, to give a total score of 0–10 at each time (Table 19.1). The score cannot be used to determine the need for resuscitation or other treatment, which should be given on clinical grounds. Depression of the score may occur because of factors other than perinatal asphyxia, including gestational age, maternal medications and congenital anomalies. In premature neonates

Table 19.1 The Apgar scoring system

Sign	0	1	2
Heart rate (per min)	Absent	< 100	> 100
Respiratory effort	Absent	Weak cry	Strong cry
Muscle tone	Limp	Some flexion	Good flexion
Reflex irritability to pharyngeal suction	None	Some motion	Cry
Colour	Central cyanosis or pallor	Centrally pink, peripheral cyanosis	Pink

the score is affected more by gestational age than by asphyxia, and premature neonates in optimal condition usually have a lower score than term neonates in optimal condition. Although in term neonates there is a good relationship between severe depression of the Apgar scores (0–3) and risk of death or handicap, in general the score is insensitive and non-specific at predicting long-term outcome for the neonate.

2. Meconium-stained amniotic fluid is seen most commonly in term and post-term neonates in whom asphyxia prior to birth stimulates intestinal peristalsis and relaxation of the anal sphincter. Heavy meconium staining of amniotic fluid is considered to be a marker of a significant asphyxial episode, although the majority of neonates with this condition do well with appropriate resuscitation and treatment. Meconium aspiration is a common cause of neonatal morbidity, and about 10 per cent of deliveries involve meconium in the amniotic fluid. Over 50 per cent of these cases have meconium in the trachea, but only around 20 per cent develop respiratory disease. Meconium aspiration may cause aspiration pneumonia, respiratory distress, pneumothorax and persistent foetal circulation with pulmonary hypertension. Ideally, if meconium staining is detected during labour, delivery should occur in stages to allow suction of the neonate's mouth, nose and pharynx before the first breath. The fact that meconium is still found in the trachea of many neonates with meconium-stained amniotic fluid even if these precautions are taken suggests the occurrence of intrauterine aspiration. After delivery the child is dried and placed in a warm resuscitation incubator and the pharynx is visualized with a laryngoscope to allow any visible meconium to be sucked out. If meconium is visible below the vocal cords, the trachea is then intubated and the lower airways suctioned.

3. Around 1 per cent of all new-born infants require resuscitation involving artificial ventilation, and 0.5 per cent of term neonates require endotracheal intubation. Reasons for this include significant prematurity, meconium aspiration, maternal illness, effects of anaesthetic or analgesic drugs administered to the mother, and congenital abnormalities. The interventions required, in order of frequency, are simple supportive measures such as drying and warming the neonate, suction of the mouth and gentle stimulation. Neonates who fail to respond to these measures require oxygen and ventilation with a bag and mask. In the event that these are inadequate external cardiac massage is required, and small numbers of neonates require drug administration. It is important that the response to each treatment is assessed before more aggressive treatments are given, in order to avoid unnecessary interventions and potential complications.

Quickly drying the neonate and placing him or her under a radiant heater on the resuscitation trolley with an integral overhead heater can reduce heat loss. Stimulation of the child should be gentle, and involves rubbing the back or tickling the feet. If suctioning is required to clear the airway, the mouth should be cleared before the nose. In the event of possible meconium aspiration, the trachea should be suctioned under direct vision before other resuscitation measures are taken. Suction should be gentle, bearing in mind that stimulation of the oropharynx can initiate a vagal response with bradycardia or apnoea. Suction attempts should be limited to 3–5 s, and the heart rate monitored during them. Spontaneous or assisted ventilation with 100 per cent oxygen should occur between attempts.

The above measures should take only a few seconds and allow assessment of respiratory effort. If effective spontaneous ventilation is not established after 10 seconds, or if the heart rate is less than 100 beats per minute, then intermittent positive pressure ventilation of the neonate with 100 per cent oxygen is required. Ventilation is also required if respirations are gasping or ineffective, or if there is persisting central cyanosis despite the administration of supplementary oxygen. This may be provided using a T-piece or a self-inflating bag. The T-piece requires expertise but is more flexible and comfortable to use, while the self-inflating bag can be used by any doctor or midwife. Self-inflating bags usually have a pressure-limiting valve that opens at 35–40 cm H_2O, which may be inadequate for the initial breaths of a neonate. For this reason, it should be possible to adjust or bypass this valve if necessary. Effective ventilation using a facemask is more important initially than endotracheal intubation. If the infant has never breathed, then the initial breaths administered will require high pressures of 30–60 cm H_2O to overcome surface tension forces within the alveoli and expand the lungs. Once this is done, lower pressures of 20–30 cm H_2O are usually adequate with a rate of 40–60 breaths per minute. Adequate chest wall movement is the best indicator of adequate inflation pressures. If ventilation is ineffective despite high inflation pressures, the airway will need to be adjusted by repositioning the head and the facemask. Over-extension of the neck may occlude the airway. If the stomach becomes distended, an oro-gastric tube should be passed and aspirated. If after 15–30 s of ventilation the heart rate has increased and colour improved, then ventilation may be reduced and withdrawn if tolerated by the child. In the event of no improvement or the reduction in ventilation compromising the child, then endotracheal intubation should be performed. This controls the airway and allows controlled ventilation with high inspired concen-trations of oxygen. A size 2.5-, 3.0- or 3.5-mm parallel-sided endotracheal tube is used, depending on the gestation and weight of the child, and most resuscitation trolleys have a chart suggesting suitable sizes and lengths of tube. Tapered endotracheal tubes may cause subglottic stenosis and are no longer used. Correct placement is indicated by observation of symmetrical chest movements, equal bilateral breath sounds with absent sounds in the stomach, and capnography if available.

If the heart rate remains below 60 beats per minute or is between 60 and 80 but not increasing despite effective ventila-tion with 100 per cent oxygen, then external cardiac massage should be instituted. Chest compression may be performed by placing the two thumbs in the middle third of the sternum and encircling the torso and supporting the back with the hands. The thumbs lie side by side on the sternum just below the nipple line. Alternatively, two-finger compression may be performed with the first and second fingers of one hand on the sternum just below the nipple line, with the other hand supporting the child's back. The sternum is com-pressed 1–3 cm, depending on the size of the child, at a rate of 120 compressions per minute. Compressions should be smooth and occupy 50 per cent of each cycle.

If the child's condition does not improve with effective ventilation and external cardiac massage, then drug administration is indicated. Routes of access include the umbilical vein (taking care to avoid positioning an intrahepatic catheter tip in the portal vein) or a peripheral vein if these can be cannulated without undue delay. There is little experience with the intraosseous route of administration in neonates, and this should be avoided if other routes are available. Endotracheal administration of drugs in 3–5 ml of normal saline can be used for adrenaline and naloxone, using the same doses as for intravenous administration, although the efficacy of this is unclear. Adrenaline is indicated for bradycardia or asystole in a dose of 10 μg/kg (0.1 ml/kg of 1/10 000 solution) flushed through the cannula with saline. Volume administration is indicated for evidence of perinatal haemorrhage indicated by pallor despite oxygenation, faint pulses with a good heart rate and poor response to resuscitation. Blood, plasma or crystalloid in aliquots of 10 ml/kg repeated as necessary according to response are used. Naloxone in a dose of 10 μg/kg is indicated if the mother has been chronically exposed to opioids during pregnancy, or given them in hospital within 4 hours of delivery. If the child is demonstrated to be acidotic by analysis of a capillary blood gas, or this is suspected on clinical grounds, then sodium bicarbonate 1–2 mmol/kg as a 4.2% solution (2–4 ml/kg) may be given intravenously followed by a flush of saline.

Once the acute phase of resuscitation is over, ongoing care of the child should begin with:

a. Provision of a warm environment in a neonatal incubator with temperature measurement
b. A chest radiograph to determine the position of the endotracheal tube
c. Measurement of plasma glucose and treatment of hypoglycaemia
d. Arterial or capillary gas analysis to guide optimization of ventilation and treatment of acidosis
e. Obtaining secure vascular access
f. Optimization of cardiac output and perfusion with volume or inotropes if required
g. Completion of documentation associated with resuscitation and treatment of the child.

Once the child is stable, transfer to a special care baby unit should be arranged.

Key learning points

- The APGAR score is a rapid and useful assessment upon which to base interventions, and is of short-term prognostic value.
- Remove meconium from the mouth and airways before ventilating the baby if at all possible.
- Neonatal resuscitation priorities are also ABC (Airway, Breathing, Circulation).

Further reading

McINTOSH, N. (1998). The newborn. In: *Forfar and Arneil's Textbook of Pediatrics*, 5th edn (A. G. M Campbell and I. McIntosh, eds), Ch. 5, pp. 113–38. Churchill Livingstone.
ZIDEMAN, D. A. (1997). Paediatric and neonatal life support. *Br. J. Anaesth.*, **79**, 178–87.

Case 20

A 7-year-old boy presents for a living related donor renal transplant. The child suffered haemolytic uraemic syndrome 5 years ago, and developed end-stage renal failure after this. He currently undergoes continuous ambulatory peritoneal dialysis, receives nocturnal feeding supplements by nasogastric tube, and has been on the waiting list for a cadaveric transplant for 3 years. The donor is his father. The child weighs 17 kg. Full blood count is: Hb, 10.7 g/dl; WBC, 8.7×10^9/l; platelets, 238×10^9/l. Electrolytes are: sodium, 137 mmol/l; potassium, 5.4 mmol/l; urea, 17.6 mmol/l; creatinine, 445 μmol/l; chloride, 110 mmol/l.

Questions

1. What is the aetiology of chronic renal failure in children?
2. What are the manifestations of chronic renal failure in children?
3. What are the principles of treating this condition?
4. Outline the anaesthetic management of this patient.

80

Answers

1. The commonest causes of end-stage renal failure in children in the developed world are congenital and hereditary conditions (reflux nephropathy, polycystic kidneys, hypoplasia and dysplasia, posterior urethral valves) in 60–65 per cent and acquired conditions (glomerulonephritis, haemolytic uraemic syndrome) in 35–40 per cent of cases. There is an incidence of two to five per million children requiring renal replacement therapy in the UK. A glomerular filtration rate of less than 50 ml/min per 1.73 m^2 is associated with a number of metabolic abnormalities. Progressive growth failure occurs at a glomerular filtration rate of less than 25 ml/min per 1.73m^2, and renal replacement therapy is required when the glomerular filtration rate is less than 10 ml/min per 1.73 m^2.

2. The main manifestations of chronic renal failure are growth failure caused by acidosis, sodium depletion, renal osteodystrophy, and inadequate calorie intake. Renal osteodystrophy is a consequence of hypocalcaemia, phosphate retention, secondary hyperparathyroidism and skeletal resistance to parathyroid hormone. Anaemia is secondary to inadequate production of erythropoietin. Platelets are usually normal in number and life span, but function may be impaired. Hypertension occurs secondary to fluid overload or alterations in the renin–angiotensin–aldosterone system. There will also be a considerable psychological burden for the child and his family, associated with chronic ill health, the requirement for frequent hospital visits and intensive medical treatment, the distress of repeated venepunctures and uncertainty about long-term prognosis.

3. Acidosis may need to be corrected with sodium bicarbonate. Depending on the manifestations of the disease, salt supplementation is necessary in cases with polyuria and sodium wasting, while children with salt and water retention will require sodium and water restriction. Measures to treat renal osteodystrophy include 1α-hydroxycholecalciferol, phosphate restriction, and calcium carbonate to bind phosphate. Erythropoietin may be given to treat anaemia, but this is limited by concerns about worsening hypertension. Growth hormone is known to be effective, but is not currently widely used because it may increase renal plasma flow, produce glomerular hyperfiltration and worsen renal function. Nutritional supplements to provide energy and sustain growth are usually required.

The definitive treatment of choice is a renal transplant. Peritoneal dialysis and haemodialysis provide incomplete renal replacement, and are considered inferior to transplantation in most cases. Renal transplant patients have a better survival than do dialysis patients of the same age, and there are psychological benefits associated with independence and freedom from dialysis. Cadaveric paediatric kidneys are a very scarce resource, and the use of living related donors allows planned elective transplantation from a donor with a good haplotype match. These have better short- and long-term graft survival rates than cadaveric grafts. One-year survival rates in the UK are 80 per cent for cadaveric grafts and over 90 per cent for live donor transplants. In children, vascular anastomoses to the aorta and inferior vena cava are often performed in preference to anastomoses to the iliac vessels.

4. Since this an elective procedure, the condition of the recipient can be optimized prior to surgery. The patient should have undergone recent dialysis and have normal electrolytes and haemoglobin and not be hypervolaemic. Antihypertensive medication should be continued until the time of surgery. Patients should be fasted in the normal way, and premedicated if appropriate. Anaesthesia can be induced intravenously or by inhalation. A rapid sequence induction is sometimes performed if there are concerns about the delayed gastric emptying associated with renal failure. Many anaesthetists prefer not to use suxamethonium because of the increase in plasma potassium that it produces. The trachea is intubated and ventilation controlled. Anaesthesia is maintained with a volatile agent in oxygen, and nitrous oxide is usually omitted to prevent distension of the bowel, which may make abdominal closure difficult. A neuromuscular relaxant that does not depend on renal elimination is used, and an infusion of atracurium of 0.5 mg/kg per hour is suitable. Analgesia is required, and fentanyl is the most widely used opioid since no active metabolites are excreted by the kidneys. Monitoring consists of ECG, non-invasive blood pressure, pulse oximetry, capnography, the degree of neuromuscular blockade, and inspired oxygen and volatile agent concentration. Temperature should be measured, along with central venous pressure and urine production from a urinary catheter. An arterial line may be sited, particularly if the child may have the aorta cross-clamped, but these are not routinely used in case a future arteriovenous shunt is required. Fluids are administered to

maintain slight hypervolaemia with a CVP of 10–12 cm H_2O and a stable blood pressure. Electrolyte and glucose concentrations should be measured during the procedure to determine the most appropriate fluids for administration. Irradiated blood should be used and given through a white cell filter if transfusion is required. Reperfusion of a large, cold, ischaemic adult kidney when the vascular clamps are removed may result in hypovolaemia and hypotension, and this should be prevented by administration of a bolus of colloid (10–20 ml/kg) just before the clamps are released Cross-clamping of the aorta may have the same effect when the clamp is released, and rapid volume administration may be required. Antibiotics, immunosuppressants, diuretics and inotropes are administered according to the locally agreed protocols.

At the end of the procedure, neuromuscular blockade should be reversed and the child extubated awake. In children of less than 20 kg respiration is occasionally compromised by the presence of an adult kidney in the abdomen, and supplementary oxygen may be required. Fluids are administered to replace hourly urine output, with an allowance of about 10 ml/kg per 24 hours for insensible losses. This regimen is adjusted in the light of central venous pressure, and the electrolyte content of the fluids is varied according to frequent measurements of plasma electrolytes. Postoperative analgesia may be provided by an intravenous infusion of opioid such as morphine sulphate (10–40 μg/kg per hour). There are advantages to using patient-controlled analgesia in older children who have had adequate preoperative instruction (bolus dose 20 μg/kg; lockout interval 5 minutes) because, if used appropriately, this titrates opioid administration to requirements and takes account of impaired metabolism or excretion of opioids. In younger children, nurse-controlled analgesia (bolus dose 40 μg/kg, infusion 10 μg/kg per hour, lockout interval 20 minutes) may be more effective and flexible than a simple infusion of morphine. Non-steroidal agents are not used, but there are no contraindications to paracetamol. Epidural techniques may be used, but some anaesthetists are concerned about a coagulopathy from impaired platelet function and the intraoperative administration of heparin.

Key learning points

- The causes of chronic renal failure in children are congenital in two-thirds and acquired in one-third of cases.
- Living related donor transplantation is becoming more common due to a shortage of cadaveric organs for transplantation.

Further reading

ALLEN, R. D. M. and CHAPMAN, J. R. (1994). *A Manual of Renal Transplantation*. Edward Arnold.
WATSON, A. R. (1998). Disorders of the urinary system. In: *Forfar and Arneil's Textbook of Pediatrics*, 5th edn (A. G. M Campbell and I. McIntosh), Ch. 17, pp. 934–84. Churchill Livingstone.

Case 21

A 12-year-old African girl is admitted to Accident & Emergency complaining of severe knee pain. She is known to have sickle cell disease, and has no history of injuring her knee.

Questions

1. What is the most likely cause of her pain?
2. Outline a plan for managing the situation.

Answers

1. Sickle cell disease is a significant problem in both Africa and the USA, affecting approximately 1 in 600 of African-Americans. An acute 'crisis' causing a discrete episode of pain is the most frequent reason for hospital admission, and this would be the most likely cause of the girl's pain. The abnormal haemoglobin – haemoglobin S – results from the substitution of a valine molecule for a glutamate in position 6 of the beta chain. This altered haemoglobin readily forms polymers when deoxygenated, producing the pathognomonic sickled

red blood cells. If a large number of these cells aggregate and adhere to the capillary endothelium then blood flow is occluded, with potential tissue ischaemia and necrosis. This will be perceived as pain if the area is large enough and contains nociceptors. The majority of painful episodes occur without a precipitating factor. Sickle cell pain ranges through the spectrum from acute to chronic, and is unpredictable in its timing, location and intensity. Although it may be as severe as that due to a malignancy, life expectancy is very different and analgesic regimens should take this into account.

2. When considering a plan of management for this girl, there are a number of factors that need to be taken into account. It is likely that she has suffered several painful episodes due to the disease, and may therefore be well known to the paediatric service. Ideally she would already have an analgesic plan available for consultation on admission. Her own past experiences and those of the family, along with the involvement of a multi-disciplinary team, are further features, and may influence whether the girl has inpatient treatment or goes home. Pharmacological intervention is the mainstay of therapy for the acute episode. The analgesic ladder approach recommended by the World Health Organization for the treatment of cancer pain is applicable to the management of sickle cell pain. Simple analgesics such as paracetamol and the non-steroidal anti-inflammatory drugs (NSAIDs) are given first on a PRN basis, and then timed regularly for moderate pain. Sickle cell disease produces the only common pain syndrome in which opioids are considered the major therapy and are started in early childhood and continued throughout adult life. As this girl is 12 years old and has severe pain, PCA (patient-controlled analgesia) is an appropriate way of administering systemic opiates to control the pain of the acute episode. This should be in conjunction with adjuvant simple analgesia, and supervised carefully. Morphine is the drug usually tried first. Parameters for PCA often need to be different in sickle cell pain than postoperative or cancer pain. A large bolus dose with a short lock-out time is often required to gain control in the initial stages, especially as these patients may be opioid tolerant. If a background infusion is also used, there should be close patient observation in case the pain abates quickly and excessive sedation results. Opioid tolerance resulting in addiction is obviously a concern in those involved with this particular patient group, but this should not preclude the child from receiving an appropriate dose of opiate. Often the

child develops a preference for a particular analgesic drug, and this should be taken into account. The aim of therapy is to return the girl to as normal an existence as possible and minimize disruption to school and social life. The multidisciplinary team and community support services have an important role in this respect.

Key learning points

- Patient-controlled analgesia is the technique of choice for severe sickle cell crises.
- A multidisciplinary approach is the most effective way of managing these cases.

Further reading

BALLAS, S. K. (1998). *Sickle cell pain. Progrress in Pain Research and Management*, Vol. 11. IASP Press.

ESSELTINE, D. W. and BAXTER, M. R. N. (1988). Sickle cell states and the anaesthetist. *Can. J. Anaesth.*, **35(4),** 385–403.

JACOBSON, S. J., KOPECKY, E. A., PRASHANT, J. and BABUL, N. (1997). Randomised trial of oral morphine for painful episodes of sickle-cell disease in children. *Lancet,* **350,** 1358–61.

PAYNE, R. (1997). Pain management in sickle cell anaemia. *Anesthesiol. Clin. North Am.*, **15(2),** 305–18.

Case 22

A 9-year-old boy with severe eczema and asthma is scheduled for inguinal hernia repair. He is currently taking steroid and beta-2 agonist inhalers for his asthma control, and has recently completed a course of oral prednisolone. He is also prescribed hydrocortisone cream for his eczema.

Questions

1. What are the potential problems when a child receiving steroid therapy undergoes anaesthesia and surgery?

2. What precautions are necessary to prevent these problems occurring?
3. Which other paediatric patient groups are likely to receive steroid therapy during treatment?

Answers

1. When a child receives exogenous glucocorticoid therapy, there is a potential for suppression of pituitary-adrenal function as with the adult patient. In the normal child, surgical stimulation is known to produce an immediate 'stress response', with the resultant secretion of anterior and posterior pituitary hormones. One of these, ACTH (corticotrophin) is produced in the anterior part of the pituitary and results in a consequent increase in plasma cortisol from the adrenal gland. Cortisol has the effects of glucose, lipid and protein mobilization, in addition to fluid retention. Whilst these functions may have been invaluable as an aid to survival in the injured or surgically traumatized patient in the past, modern techniques of anaesthesia and perioperative care may render the rise in cortisol less crucial. There is still the risk, however, that the child receiving steroid treatment by whatever route has a degree of adrenal suppression. If he cannot mount a sufficient cortisol response to surgery he has the potential to develop an 'Addisonian crisis', with resultant hypotension and cardiovascular instability. If a child requires permanent replacement steroid therapy due to a non-functioning adrenal gland, this is given in a dosage regimen of around 10 mg/m^2. In addition, the other side effects of long-term steroid therapy may be apparent. In children there is concern about bone growth, they may be Cushingoid and overweight and have impaired wound healing associated with immunosuppression.
2. When presented with this case, the first question to ask is, does the child require any additional dose of steroid to cover his perioperative period? This depends on the daily dose he is getting through his various therapies. It is important to question his parents as to when exactly the course of prednisolone ended and how often he uses his steroid inhalers. Recent recommendations for adults have suggested that after a course of prednisolone, a 3-month interval should have elapsed to ensure normal functioning of the hypothalamic-pituitary axis.

There is little similar information available in paediatric practice specific to the perioperative period. However, the '3-month safety period' would seem to be a reasonable guideline. The dose of steroid administered in the hydrocortisone cream is dependent on the sites and surface area of the body to which it is applied, as well as to the strength and frequency with which it is administered. It important to establish the exact nature of the preparation, as parents are sometimes unaware of its implications. The only way to definitively diagnose adrenal suppression is to test the function of the hypothalamic–pituitary axis with stimulation tests. Random single-serum cortisol measurements are inadequate. Requirement for steroid supplementation is obviously dependent on the degree of surgical stress that the patient will undergo, and it may be that the hernia repair does not generate a marked stress response. Previous regimens have recommended 'supraphysiological' doses of steroid therapy. This seems unnecessary, given that cortisol levels usually return to normal in 24 hours after moderate surgery. The high doses given may themselves cause deleterious effects with regard to wound healing and blood glucose control, and steroid supplementation should therefore not be given as a matter of course. If a child is undergoing a major surgical procedure and has known adrenal suppression, it is recommended to use two to three times their normal steroid dose during the first 24 hours, tailoring by 50 per cent increments over the next 5 days until they are back to their original regimen.

3. Other situations where children receiving steroids come to surgery are those with congenital adrenal hyperplasia, renal patients (e.g. with nephrotic syndrome), and patients on immunosuppressive doses of steroids after organ transplantation or in the treatment of malignancy. Those with congenital adrenal hyperplasia are often having major corrective surgery of anatomical abnormalities, and require mineralocorticoid replacement in addition to the glucocorticoids. The use of epidural anaesthesia for such cases may decrease the perioperative stress response. If a child is on steroid immunosuppression, it is mandatory to continue the equivalent steroid dose throughout (Table 22.1). Additional steroids are not, however, required, as the doses used are sufficient to maintain cardiovascular stability.

Table 22.1 Table showing equivalent anti-inflammatory doses of glucocorticoids

Drug	Equivalent anti-inflammatory doses (mg)
Betamethasone	0.75
Cortisone acetate	25
Dexamethasone	0.75
Hydrocortisone	20
Methylprednisolone	4
Prednisolone	5
Prednisone	5
Triamcinolone	4

Key learning point

- The 3-month safety period is a reasonable guideline for peri-operative steroid supplementation.

Further reading

BRITISH NATIONAL FORMULARY (1999). Section 6.3: Corticosteroids, **37**, 316–17.
NICHOLSON, G., BURRIN, J. M. and HALL, G. M. (1998). Perioperative steroid supplemenation. *Anaesthesia*, **53**, 1091–1104.
WOLF, A .R., EYERS, R. L., LAUSSEN, P. C. *et al.* (1993). Effect of epidural anaesthesia on stress responses to abdominal surgery in infants. *Br. J. Anaesth.*, **70(6)**, 654–60.

Case 23

A 6-month-old Down's syndrome baby presents to the Accident & Emergency department in a collapsed state. The mother gives a 24-hour history of pallor, sweating and lethargy associated with poor feeding and rapid, noisy breathing. The baby had undergone an uneventful closure of an atrioventricular canal defect 1 month previously. Since discharge from hospital the baby had been well. On examination the baby is cool peripherally with a capillary refill time of 5 s. There is a palpable liver edge of 4 cm, and the heart rate is noted to be 240 beats per minute with narrow and regular QRS complexes.

Questions

1. What is the provisional diagnosis?
2. What are the ECG characteristics of this dysrhythmia?
3. What are the potential causes of this dysrhythmia?
4. What investigations do you require to investigate this baby fully?
5. How do you treat this dysrhythmia?

Answers

1. The provisional diagnosis is of supraventricular tachycardia (SVT) associated with cardiac failure. SVT is the commonest sustained dysrhythmia in the paediatric population, occurring most frequently in neonates and infants. Although not immediately life threatening, if not treated it can lead to cardiovascular collapse and clinical evidence of shock. In approximately 90 per cent of SVTs the mechanism of origin is one of a re-entry circuit, which may occur at the AV node, the SA node, or via the atrial muscle. Occasionally it may be due to an accessory connection, as with Wolff–Parkinson–White syndrome, where there is an accessory bundle of Kent. The remaining 5–10 per cent of SVTs are caused by enhanced automaticity.

2. SVT is usually a rapid and regular dysrhythmia. The heart rate obviously varies with the age of the infant, but is usually greater than 230 beats per minute. AV block is usually a rare finding in SVT, so the rhythm is invariably regular. If the ventricular rate is very fast, P waves may not be evident. The QRS complexes are of normal duration, i.e. < 0.08 s. SVTs with wide complexes due to aberrant conduction are very rare, and can be difficult to distinguish from ventricular tachy-cardias. Occasionally, if the SVT has been sustained for a prolonged period of time, there may be signs of myocardial ischaemia with ST and T wave changes.

   It can sometimes be difficult to differentiate an SVT from a very rapid sinus tachycardia. The following points can help identify the rhythm. Normally the P wave axis, if seen, is abnormal in an SVT but normal in a sinus tachycardia. The rate may vary beat to beat with a sinus tachycardia, but this is not the case with an SVT. Finally, the heart rate is usually greater than 200 beats per minute with a sinus tachycardia, whereas the rate is usually less than 230 beats per minute with an SVT.

3. The possible causes of SVT are:

a. Congenital heart disease – ASD, AV canal defect etc.
b. Cardiomyopathy
c. Infective – myocarditis, pericarditis, pneumonia
d. Post-cardiac repair
e. Accessory bundle – Wolff–Parkinson–White syndrome
f. Drug induced – cocaine, amphetamines, antihistamines, caffeine, phenothiazines, theophylline
g. Endocrine causes – thyrotoxicosis
h. Thromboembolic – pulmonary embolism.

4. The following investigations would be required:

a. Full blood count, U & Es, glucose, calcium and magnesium
b. Twelve-lead ECG
c. CXR and echo
d. Toxicology screen if indicated
e. Thyroid function screen
f. Arterial blood gases.

5. The principles of basic life support should be instituted, i.e. A – Airway; B – Breathing; C – Circulation.

If the baby's condition is stable and there are no signs of cardiovascular collapse, the initial management should be to enhance vagal tone by using one of the following methods:

a. Diving reflex – this works by increasing vagal tone and slowing AV conduction. It is performed by wrapping the baby in a towel and immersing the whole face for 5 s. In older children it can be performed by placing an ice pack or a cloth soaked in ice-cold water over the mouth and nose.
b. Carotid sinus massage.
c. Valsalva manoeuvre.
d. Ocular pressure.

If this fails, pharmacologic management of the dysrhythmia is required. Adenosine (Adenocard) is an endogenous nucleo-side that slows the conduction time through the AV node; it has a half-life of 10 s and is the initial drug of choice. It is given as a rapid i.v. bolus of 0.1 mg/kg followed by a rapid bolus of saline 2–5 ml to avoid sequestration of the drug in red blood cells. The dose can be doubled and given again.

The maximum recommended dose is 0.25 μg/kg. Potential side effects are bronchospasm, hypotension, flushing and bradycardia. Care should be taken when administering this drug to asthmatics and children with denervated/transplanted hearts.

If the patient's condition is deteriorating and has not responded to pharmacological treatment, synchronized cardioversion is required. This is the gold standard for treatment of resistant re-entrant tachycardias. The initial energy dose required is 0.5 J/kg, and this can be doubled to 1.0 J/kg if the first shock is unsuccessful.

Once the SVT has been converted pharmacological prophylaxis will be required, as 90 per cent of SVTs will recur. In all SVTs except those due to Wolff–Parkinson–White syndrome, digoxin is the drug of choice. This drug is a cardiac glycoside, which inhibits the Na/K ATPase pump. It is given intravenously as 10 μg/kg in infants and 20 μg/kg in older children. Alternative drugs to digoxin are propranolol, verapamil, flecainide and amiodarone; these drugs require to be prescribed under the direct supervision of the paediatric cardiologist involved.

In cases of SVT which are resistant to medical therapy or those with life threatening components (e.g. Wolff–Parkinson–White syndrome), radiofrequency ablation can be used to terminate the SVT.

Key learning points

- Most SVTs in children are caused by a re-entrant mechanism.
- The heart rate is usually greater than 230 beats per minute.
- Early intervention with mechanical enhancement of vagal tone, adenosine and DC countershock are indicated to prevent a vicious cycle of clinical deterioration.
- Full investigation under the direction of a paediatric cardiologist should be arranged.

Further reading

ADVANCED LIFE SUPPORT GROUP (1993). *Advanced Paediatric Life Support*. BMJ Publishing Group.

KAMINER, S. J. and STRONG, W. B. (1994). Cardiac arrhythmias. *Paed. Rev.*, **15(11)**, 437–9.
STRASBURGER, J. F. (1991). Cardiac arrhythmias in childhood. Diagnostic considerations and treatment. *Drugs*, **42(6)**, 974–83.

Case 24

An 18-month-old boy with recurrent unilateral right-sided chest infections and persistent wheeze presents for surgical resection of a right-sided bronchogenic cyst. His weight is 13 kg. He is otherwise well, with no other relevant medical or family history. He recently underwent uneventful fibre-optic bronchoscopy.

Questions

1. Describe the anaesthetic management of this case.
2. Outline the relevant physiological changes that occur during the surgical procedure.
3. What are the options for providing postoperative analgesia for this child?

Answers

1. Review of the preoperative investigations, a recent chest film and the previous anaesthetic record is required. Blood should be cross-matched for the case. The child should be fasted for 6 hours (2 hours for clear fluids), and premedication is optional. Induction may be gaseous or intravenous after application of EMLA cream or amethocaine gel, depending on the child's veins and parental preference. After induction a secure intravenous line of adequate gauge is placed, neuromuscular relaxant administered and the child intubated with an uncuffed oral endotracheal tube. A leak should be elicited. Paediatric double-lumen tubes are rarely used, and options for isolating the lungs include endobronchial intubation with an uncut endotracheal tube a size smaller than would be used for normal endotracheal intubation, an endobronchial blocker

or, most commonly, relying on the surgical packs and retractors collapsing the lung and keeping it down. Appropriate monitoring comprises ECG, NIBP, central temperature, pulse oximetry, capnography, inspired oxygen concentration and inspired volatile agent concentration. An intra-arterial line is of use for blood sampling and continuous blood pressure readings, but is not essential.

Maintenance of anesthesia is with a volatile agent in oxygen and air or oxygen and nitrous oxide. An opioid such as morphine sulphate 0.1–0.2 mg/kg or fentanyl 5 μg/kg per hour is usually given. The inspired oxygen concentration is adjusted to produce an adequate arterial oxygen saturation, and the application of positive end expiratory pressure may help with this while the upper lung is collapsed. Neuromuscular blockade and intermittent positive pressure ventilation are required. In a healthy child who has not undergone extensive lung resection, reversal of anaesthesia and extubation should be the norm. A chest drain is placed by the surgeon and hand bagging performed during chest closure to eliminate the residual pneumothorax. Anaesthesia is discontinued, the neuromuscular blockade reversed, the trachea suctioned via the endotracheal tube, the pharynx suctioned and the child extubated when breathing adequately and awake.

2. Thoracic surgery is normally performed in the lateral position, which has implications for ventilation and perfusion of the lungs. When an awake subject lies in the lateral position, gravity causes a gradient within the thorax and perfusion is better in the dependent lung than in the upper one. The dependent lung occupies a more favourable position on the pulmonary compliance curve, and the diaphragm on that side is pushed higher by the weight of the abdominal contents. As a result it contracts more efficiently. These effects mean that ventilation and perfusion are well matched under these circumstances and there is little increase in shunt. In an anaesthetized patient in the lateral position, perfusion remains better in the dependent lung but the distribution of ventilation is altered. There is a loss of functional residual capacity and a reduction in compliance of the lungs. The dependent lung now occupies a less favourable position on the compliance curve than the upper lung, and ventilation is preferentially distributed to the upper lung. A ventilation–perfusion mismatch develops, with a decrease in the arterial oxygen tension. When the thorax is open during surgery these changes are exacerbated, and the use of relaxants and intermittent positive

pressure ventilation results in an overventilated, under-perfused upper lung and an overperfused, underventilated lower lung. Collapse of the upper lung during surgery tends to redistribute ventilation to the better-perfused lower lung so that the dependent lung now receives the entire minute ventilation, but because the upper lung is still perfused the intrapulmonary shunt tends to increase further under these circumstances.

3. After major surgery it is difficult to provide adequate analgesia without adverse effects using only one analgesic modality. Ideally the child should receive a combination of analgesic drugs to improve efficacy and minimize the side effects of any one kind of analgesic. Opioid may be administered by intravenous infusion, nurse-controlled analgesia, intermittent intravenous boluses or via the epidural route. The local anaes-thetic technique may be intercostal nerve blocks performed percutaneously by the anaesthetist or under direct vision by the surgeon. If they are performed by the surgeon, then an epi-dural catheter may also be placed in either the paravertebral region or in the interpleural space to permit a continuous infu-sion or top-ups with a local anaesthetic solution. Alternatively, a standard intervertebral epidural may be performed to place the tip of the catheter in the centre of the nerve roots that supply the dermatomes involved in the surgery. If there are no contraindications, regular administration of a non-steroidal anti-inflammatory agent will reduce the requirements for opioid and local anaesthetic and improve the efficacy of the analgesic technique.

If intercostal nerve blocks are performed with 0.5% bupiva-caine + adrenaline 1/200 000, an opioid will also be required for pain not covered by the blocks and for when they regress. This could be an intravenous infusion of morphine sulphate (10–40 μg/kg per hour). Nurse-controlled analgesia (bolus dose 20–40 μg/kg, infusion 10–20 μg/kg per hour, lockout interval 20–30 minutes) may be more effective and flexible than a simple infusion. If a catheter is left in the paravertebral or the interpleural space, then an infusion or intermittent top-ups with bupivacaine (maximum dose 0.25 mg/kg per hour) will reduce the requirement for opioid. For an epidural infu-sion, bupivacaine 0.125% with fentanyl 1–2 μg/ml infused at a rate not exceeding 0.375 mg/kg per hour of bupivacaine may be used. Alternatively, an epidural infusion of bupivacaine 0.125% alone can be used with an intravenous infusion of morphine sulphate (10–40 μg/kg per hour). Oral analgesics may be added after 24–48 hours, when the child is able to absorb them and when the requirement for potent system analgesia is reducing. Co-analgesia with NSAIDs and para-cetamol is particularly helpful. Removal of the chest drain(s) will require some supplementary analgesia, and the nature of this will depend on what analgesia the child is already receiving. A simple intravenous bolus of morphine sulphate (50–100 μg/kg) will be adequate. Alternatively, an epidural top-up or top-up of an intervertebral or interpleural catheter may be performed. Another option is inhaled nitrous oxide.

Key learning points

- As thoracic surgery is usually performed in the lateral position, careful consideration should be given to ventilation/perfusion matching.
- Multimodal analgesia is very effective after paediatric thoracic surgery.

Further reading

CHEUNG, S. L. W., BOOKER, P. D., FRANKS, R. and POZZI, M. (1997). Serum concentrations of bupivacaine during prolonged continuous paravertebral infusion in young infants. *Br. J. Anaesth.*, **79**, 9–13.

KARMAKAR, M. K., BOOKER, P. D., FRANKS, R. and POZZI, M. (1996). Continuous extra-pleural paravertebral infusion of bupivacaine for post-thoracotomy analgesia in young infants. *Br. J. Anaesth.*, **76**, 811–15.

MORRAY, J. P., KRANE, E. J., GEIDUSCHEK, J. M. and O'ROURKE, P. P. (1994). Anesthesia for thoracic surgery. In: *Pediatric Anesthesia* (G. A. Gregory, ed.), Ch. 15, 421–64. Churchill Livingstone.

Case 25

A 12-year-old girl presents to your hospital. She has been pyrexial for 24 hours, and this has been associated with poor appetite and intermittent abdominal pain. In addition, she has been dyspnoeic with a dry cough. On history taking, you discover that she suffers from cystic fibrosis and 1 year ago under went double lung trans-plantation for end-stage respiratory failure. Her vital signs are stable, with a BP of 110/75, heart rate of 120/min and a respiratory rate of 22/min. On further questioning, you find that she has had only one episode of acute rejection since the transplant and this was approximately 3 months ago. On this occasion she required an increase in her steroid therapy as well as a short course of OKT3.

Questions

1. How are you able to differentiate acute rejection from an episode of infection?
2. What types of immunosuppressive therapy are there, and what are their well-recognized side effects? How will the immuno-suppressive therapy influence your anaesthetic management of this patient?
3. What are the physiological implications of lung transplantation, and how will this affect your anaesthetic?
4. The general surgeon has decided that this girl has acute appendicitis and requires to go to theatre for appendicectomy. What are the other potential causes of acute abdomen in this girl's case?
5. What are the important aspects of anaesthetizing a post-transplant patient?

Answers

1. Differentiating between acute rejection and acute infection can be difficult; however, it is vitally important to make the diagnosis, as the treatment regimens are completely different. Acute rejection is most likely to occur in the first 3 months following the transplant. The patient will commonly present with a cough, pyrexia and breathlessness, and these symptoms will be associated frequently with lung infiltrates on chest X-ray.
   The clinical criteria for diagnosis of acute rejection are:

   a. Temperature: increase $> 0.5\,°C$ above baseline.
   b. P_aO_2 decrease > 10 mmHg below baseline.
   c. Radiology: new or changing infiltrates.
   d. Spirometry: decrease in $FEV_1 > 10$ per cent below baseline.
   e. Infection excluded.
   f. Response to treatment with corticosteroids.

The symptoms are non-specific and could well be indicators of infection, especially in this child with a background of cystic fibrosis. The diagnosis of rejection is aided by transbronchial biopsy and bronchio-alveolar lavage. Sometimes the response to steroids is used to differentiate between the two conditions.

2. Most transplant patients will be maintained on a triple therapy regimen consisting of cyclosporine A, azothioprine and corticosteroids, and it is imperative that the administration of these drugs is continued and not abruptly stopped. If the oral route of administration is not possible due to ongoing intra-abdominal pathology, the immunosuppressive therapy must be given intravenously. The transplant centre involved will give advice on immunosuppressive therapy.

Cyclosporine A is a cyclic peptide derived from fungus, which suppresses cytotoxic T-cell development and B-cell function. Its major side effects are of nephrotoxicity, hepato-toxicity, hypertension and neurological sequelae (e.g. tremors and seizures). Gastric atony can also occur, and will obviously influence the type of anaesthetic the child is given. Meto-clopramide is known to be effective in treating this side effect. Electrolyte imbalances also occur – for example, hyper-kaleamia and hypomagnesaemia. Cyclosporine A has a very narrow therapeutic window, so drugs that induce or inhibit its metabolism by cytochrome P450 will affect its drug level. It is also known to enhance the duration of action of neuro-muscular blockers such as vecuronium and atracurium. The effects of drugs like fentanyl and thiopentone have been shown to be enhanced when administered concurrently with cyclosporine.

Azothioprine is an antimetabolite that blocks DNA/RNA synthesis. Bone marrow depression occurs commonly with its use. Hepatotoxicity as well as pancreatitis can also occur. Due to its inhibitory action on phosphodiesterase, the action of suxamethonium may be prolonged and its effect on non-depolarizers can be unpredictable.

Corticosteroids have well recognized side effects of oedema, hypertension, peptic ulceration, hypokalaemia, hypo-calcaemia and glucose intolerance.

OKT3 and antilymphocyte globulin are used to treat cases of acute rejection that are not responding to high dose steroids. They may also be part of the maintenance regimen. Side effects include arthralgia, leucopenia and thrombocytopenia. OKT3 can also produce signs of non-cardiogenic pulmonary oedema and hypotension, as well as nausea and vomiting.

When a post-transplant patient requires anaesthesia, it is important to be aware of the side effects of these immuno-suppressive drugs. Therefore, the anaesthetist's preoperative assessment should include a full blood count to assess bone marrow function and evidence of infection, and U&Es and LFTs to look for impaired renal and liver function along with electrolyte imbalance.

3. The physiological consequences of lung transplantation are due to the disruption in the nerve supply, lymphatic supply and blood supply to the donor lungs. In addition, there may be disruption to the nerve supply to the donor heart.

The donor lungs are effectively denervated from the level of the anastamosis downwards. With sequential trans-plantations, this is at the level of the bronchi. The airway distal to the anastamosis will not respond to stimulation; how-ever, the cough reflex is intact. In the past, lung transplants were carried out *en bloc* with a tracheal anastamosis. This meant that the airway below this level was denervated, and obviously this included the carina. The cough reflex is lost with this type of surgical approach, and the risks of infection and aspiration are increased.

Disruption of the lymphatic drainage of the lung increases the lung's extravascular water and therefore the risk of pulmonary oedema. Hypoxic vasoconstriction is maintained; however, the mucociliary clearance of the donor lung is impaired, thereby increasing the risk of infection.

If the transplantation is performed *en bloc*, the nerve supply to the native heart may be disrupted and it may therefore func-tion like a transplanted heart. As a result of loss of the auto-nomic supply, the resting heart rate is higher and there is an increased risk of developing dysrhythmias. The heart rate can only be increased by drugs with a direct beta-adrenergic action (e.g. adrenaline, isoprenaline and ephedrine). The denervated heart can only increase its cardiac output by an intrinsic Frank Starling effect, or due to the direct action of circulating catecholamines. Also the heart is very preload sensitive, and it will therefore show an increased sensitivity to hypovolaemia.

4. The cause of this girl's abdominal pain may be:

   a. Cystic fibrosis – inspissated secretions with a resulting bowel obstruction
   b. Drug-related – steroid-induced peptic ulceration, colonic perforation

c. Infection-related – cytomegalovirus can produce a gastric outlet obstruction.

5. Anaesthetizing a child who has undergone organ transplantation poses a number of challenges to the anaesthetist. The pathological process that warranted the transplant must be assessed, as well as the function of the transplanted organ. The implications of immunosuppressive therapy must be appreciated, as well as the physiological challenges of the transplant organ. Always be aware of the possibility of acute rejection.

The child must be thoroughly assessed prior to theatre; this includes a full history and background to the transplantation. The immunosuppressive therapy, along with a full drug history, must be clarified. Where required, the oral immunosuppressive agents should be converted to intravenous preparations. The Transplant Centre can and should be contacted for advice regarding the management of the child and her immunosuppression. The child should have a full physical examination, looking particularly for signs of infection/acute rejection and indicators of how well the underlying transplanted lung is functioning.

The following investigations are required as standard in order to assess the function of the transplanted organ, as well as the effects of the immunosuppressive therapy on the different organ systems: U&Es, glucose, LFTs, FBC and coagulation. Arterial blood gas analysis and CXR are required to assess the function of the transplanted lung, along with lung function tests if the patient's condition allows. On CXR, there may be signs of acute and chronic rejection (obliterative bronchiolitis). An ECG is also required, as hypertension commonly occurs due to cyclosporine A therapy.

Premedication will depend on the individual child; anxiolytics can be used provided the underlying lung function is adequate. Supplemental corticosteroids will be required, as will metoclopramide if there is a positive history of gastric atony secondary to the cyclosporine.

The importance of avoiding infection cannot be emphasized too strongly in this class of patient. These patients are prone to infection not only due to the immunosuppressive therapy, but also to their impaired defence mechanisms (i.e. abnormal mucociliary mechanism as well as the absence of the cough reflex in some cases). Antibiotic prophylaxis is required as well as an aseptic approach to the child, especially if invasive monitoring is indicated. It has been advised that nasal intubations should be avoided where possible due to the increased bacteraemia that is produced.

The type of surgery required will influence the choice of anaesthetic technique. All the induction agents and volatile agents are well tolerated. Opiates should be used carefully along with benzodiazepines as there appears to be an increased sensitivity to these drugs. Neuromuscular blocking agents can interact with the immunosuppressive therapy, and this should be taken into account when using both depolarizing and non-depolarizing agents. Local and regional anaesthesia can also be used safely in transplant patients, provided strict asepsis is adhered to.

Due to the increased risk of aspiration and the impaired protective airway reflexes, tracheal intubation is required in most cases. There is a risk of disrupting the tracheal or bronchial anastomosis if the endotracheal tube is advanced too far on intubation, and also if high airway pressures are used during intermittent positive pressure ventilation.

The response of the heart may be affected if, during transplantation, its autonomic nerve supply was disrupted. Hypovolaemia is poorly tolerated due to the heart being preload sensitive, and intraoperative bradycardias will only respond to drugs with a direct beta-agonist action. Safe anaesthesia of transplant patients can be accomplished provided the anaesthetist involved has an understanding of the altered physiology of the transplanted lung and the implications of immunosuppressive therapy.

Key learning points

- It is vital to differentiate between acute rejection and acute infection, as the treatment regimens are different.
- Immunosuppressive drug effects have important implications for the anaesthetist.

Further reading

CONACHER, I. D. (1988). Isolated lung transplantation: a review of problems and guide to anaesthesia. *Br. J. Anaesth.*, **61(4)**, 468–74.

HADDOW, G. R. (1997). Anaesthesia for patients after lung transplantation. *Can. J. Anaesth.*, **44(2)**, 182–97.

MADDEN, B. P., KAMALVAND, K., CHAN, C. M. *et al.* (1993). The medical management of patients with cystic fibrosis following heart–lung transplantation. *Eur. Resp. J.,* **6(7),** 965–70.

SHAW, I. H., KIRK, A. J. and CONACHER, I. D. (1991). Anaesthesia for patients with transplanted hearts and lungs undergoing non-cardiac surgery. *Br. J. Anaesth.,* **67(6),** 772–8.

Case 26

A 3-year-old child attended the day surgery unit for repair of an umbilical hernia. She has no significant past medical history, although her mother says she is allergic to the family cat. On examination she had a slight clear nasal discharge but no other symptoms and her chest was clear. She weighs 13 kg.

Questions

1. What factors make a child unsuitable to be treated as a day case?
2. Does this child have an upper respiratory tract infection, and what should you do about it if she does?
3. Assuming she is fit for anaesthesia, outline the anaesthetic management of the child, including a plan for analgesia.

Answers

1. Many children are appropriately managed as day cases provided they have a responsible adult to look after them following discharge. Exclusion criteria can be divided into different categories as follows:
   a. *Medical* – patients with metabolic disease such as diabetes or inborn errors of metabolism usually require assessment the night before surgery. Children with complex or untreated congenital heart disease should be managed as inpatients, and day surgery should not be undertaken if the child has an active viral or bacterial infection. Patients with well-controlled chronic disease such as asthma may be suitable if their illness is currently stable.

b. *Surgical* – procedures that are likely to take a long time and cause severe postoperative pain are unsuitable to be performed on a day case basis. If there is a high risk of postoperative haemorrhage, it also desirable to admit the child to a ward post-op.

c. *Anaesthetic* – if there is a family history of an anaesthetic problem, such as malignant hyperpyrexia, time is required for adequate preoperative preparation. Often, if the surgery takes longer than an hour or the child has a difficult airway, recovery in the ward setting is appropriate.

d. *Age* – an ex-premature baby up to 60 weeks post-conceptual age is at increased risk of postoperative apnoea following anaesthesia, and is therefore not suitable to be treated as a day case.

e. *Social* – if it is unlikely that there will be a responsible adult available at all times to look after the child in the post-operative period, then admission may be the best option. Likewise if there is a long distance for the child to travel or there is no means of private transport.

2. In order to establish whether or not this child has a respiratory tract infection, it is necessary to ask the mother about any additional symptoms such as a cough or if her child has been unwell 'in herself '. Crusting of secretions around the nares or purulent nasal secretions may give concern. The chest should be examined for signs of excessive secretions, lobar consolidation or signs of small airways disease. In this case, it is unlikely that the runny nose is caused by infection if there have been no obvious systemic symptoms or signs and the child has been generally well. Children can suffer from an average of three to eight upper respiratory tract infections (URTIs) per year, and it is often an anaesthetic dilemma as to the timing of general anaesthesia. URTIs are associated with changes in respiratory function that predispose children to laryngospasm, hypoxia, atelectasis and vagally-mediated airway hyper-reactivity. In general, if the child has a congested upper airway with infective secretions, is pyrexial or has signs of a lower respiratory tract infection, it is always safer to defer the elective procedure for 4 weeks to allow full recovery. However, many 'runny noses' are caused by an allergic rhinitis or teething, and not every child with nasal secretions needs to be cancelled.

3. A suitable anaesthetic technique for this child would begin with the application of a topical local anaesthetic such as

EMLA cream to the dorsum of both hands at least 1 hour prior to induction. Oral premedication is not usually necessary. An intravenous induction can then be performed in the presence of the mother if appropriate, using propofol (3–4 mg/kg). Anaesthesia can then be maintained using oxygen/nitrous oxide and a volatile agent such as sevoflurane or isoflurane. The airway can be secured using a laryngeal mask airway (size 2), as this is a short superficial procedure. It is advisable to ensure adequate depth of anaesthesia and to avoid intubation in this case to minimize the risk of airway irritation. Some advocate administration of atropine or glycopyrrolate to dry secretions and to counter vagally-mediated airway reflexes. Analgesia is provided using a combination of local anaesthesia plus simple analgesia, ideally avoiding the use of opiates. Local infiltration with bupivacaine (up to 2 mg/kg) can be performed at the end of the procedure by the surgeon to achieve the most accurate placement. Providing there is no history of asthma, a non-steroidal anti-inflammatory drug such as diclofenac (1 mg/kg) can be administered rectally along with paracetamol (30–40 mg/kg) at the start of the procedure. Analgesia into the postoperative period needs to be considered in paediatric day case surgery, and it is important to ensure that a regular regimen of simple analgesia has been prescribed for use at home.

Key learning points

- Pragmatic selection criteria for paediatric day case surgery should be determined locally.
- Children with URTI are more likely to suffer respiratory morbidity during and after anaesthesia.

Further reading

MARTIN, L. D. (1994). Anaesthetic implications of an upper respiratory infection in children. *Ped. Clin. North Am.*, **41,** 121–30.

MORTON, N. S. and RAINE, P. A. M. (1994). *Paediatric Day Case Surgery* Oxford University Press.

WOLF, A. R. (1999). Tears at bedtime: a pitfall of extending paediatric day-case surgery without extending analgesia. *Br. J. Anaesth.*, **82(3),** 319–20.

Case 27

A 4-year-old boy who has congenital hydrocephalus requires repair of his hypospadias. He had a ventriculo-peritoneal shunt inserted soon after birth, and had a revision of the shunt at 2 years of age due to infection. For the past 2 years, he has been well and appears to be developing normally.

Questions

1. What are the particular preoperative concerns with this patient?
2. What are the options for peri- and postoperative analgesia for a hypospadias repair in this child?
3. What techniques can be used to prolong the analgesic effect of caudal epidural blockade?

Answers

1. The main issue in this child's preoperative assessment concerns the adequate functioning of his VP shunt. In the first instance, it will be necessary to establish from his mother that he has shown no signs of raised intracranial pressure recently, such as headaches or nausea. It should also be ascertained that the boy does not suffer from any seizure activity or, if he does, that it is well under control. Any current or previous anticonvulsant medication should be documented. Clinically, the shunt can be tested to ensure it is draining CSF properly. He should also undergo a routine preoperative assessment and his previous anaesthetic charts should be reviewed. If the hydrocephalus has resulted in a large head relative to his body size, this can occasionally cause difficulty with intubation due to a prominent occiput.
2. Hypospadias occurs in approximately 1 in 500 new-borns. In the mildest cases the urethral meatus opens on the ventral aspect of the glans, but the penis may also be curved ventrally with the appearance of a dorsal hood. Surgery may be complex, and a urethral catheter is often left *in situ* for the immediate postoperative period. There is therefore a requirement for stronger and more prolonged analgesia than for a

circumcision. It is often appropriate to use local anaesthesia in a caudal epidural block, possibly in combination with a small dose of systemic opiate such as morphine. In this child, it is obviously important to confirm satisfactory VP shunt function and the absence of raised intracranial pressure before considering a regional technique. Little is known about the 'normal' ICP response to lumbar epidural injection. However, a marked rise in intracranial pressure was demonstrated in two head-injured adult patients given epidural blocks whilst they still had intracranial pressure monitoring *in situ*. This was presumably attributable to the volume (10–20 ml) and rate of injection (over 20–30 s) in patients with decreased intracranial compliance. These changes have also been demonstrated in two parturients with brain tumours who developed CNS complications after caudal analgesia, and in a porcine model. There is one report of a child with Cornelia de Lange syndrome who suffered a respiratory arrest with fixed dilated pupils after caudal injection. This syndrome features abnormal muscle tone, mental retardation and, more rarely, the possibility of seizures. One possible mechanism for the respiratory arrest (from which the child made a full recovery) was that the caudal injection had caused a marked, acute rise in intracranial pressure. In adults the dural sac ends at the level of S2, but it extends further down in children. If the sac is further distended by an increased ICP, a rapid injection into the caudal space would highlight any transmitted changes to the subarachnoid space. In view of these findings, it would therefore seem prudent to avoid epidural injections in patients with suspected increased ICP. This will not only avoid the risk of dural puncture (with potential for coning), but also acute and severe changes in ICP. In any case, with normal ICP it is recommended that the injection should be made slowly as a matter of routine to minimize any potential ICP changes.

3. The use of a 'long-acting' local anaesthetic such as bupivacaine as a single-shot caudal injection produces reliable analgesia for an average of 4 hours. The analgesic effect of the local anaesthetic can be prolonged by the use of additives or by the insertion of a catheter into the caudal space to allow top-ups of analgesia. The synergistic effect of opioids and local anaesthetics when used in the caudal epidural space is well-documented. This has been used to good effect in hypospadias repair, where a mean duration of 20 hours of analgesia was demonstrated in one study. This is due to a direct action of the opioid at the opioid receptors in the spinal cord. A signifi-

cantly smaller dose of drug is required than that needed to provide systemic analgesia. Morphine is most commonly used in a dose of around 0.03 mg/kg, and fentanyl is also used successfully. The problem with using opioids in the epidural space has always been weighing up the benefits of the analgesia against the incidence of side effects – the most severe being the risk of respiratory depression. Hypoventilation is best detected when the child is not receiving supplemental oxygen. Therefore, it is recommended that all children with opioids injected into the epidural space have continuous pulse oximetry whilst breathing air. In addition, concomitant sedative agents and systemic opioids should not be given. Opioids should not be used as additives in day case anaesthesia.

The alpha-2-adrenergic receptor agonist clonidine has also been shown significantly to prolong the analgesia when added to local anaesthetics in the caudal space in children in a dose of 1–2 μg/kg. Its action is thought to be due to stimulation of descending noradrenergic medullo-spinal pathways inhibiting the release of nociceptive neurotransmitters in the dorsal horn of the spinal cord. There appear to be no significant haemodynamic or respiratory changes associated with the use of clonidine in paediatric studies. However, the drug should probably not be used in patient groups susceptible to respiratory depression, such as neonates.

The efficacy of caudal epidural ketamine has been shown in several paediatric studies. It significantly prolongs analgesia up to four-fold when given in a dose of 0.5 mg/kg. At present there is restricted availability of preservative-free ketamine, and it is not licensed for use in the epidural space.

The addition of adrenaline to local anaesthetic has little if any effect in prolonging the analgesic effect in the epidural space. This is in contrast to the use of adrenaline-containing local anaesthetics for local infiltration.

Epidural catheters can be inserted into the epidural space via the sacral hiatus, either by threading the catheter through a cannula or by using a 5-cm Tuohy needle. There are now specially designed 'caudal catheter' packs, which incorporate a thin stylette inside the catheter in order to facilitate threading the catheter into the space. The catheter can then be secured for repeated use in order to provide postoperative analgesia. The risk of contamination from the perianal area is minimized if meticulous attention is paid to aseptic technique, the entrance site is covered with a sterile dressing, and the catheter is removed after 48 hours. Continuous-infusion epidural analgesia for hypospadias correction is probably the analgesic technique of choice, and is also very effective in preventing bladder spasms. Should these occur, however, antispasmodic treatment with oxybutinin or the benzodiazepines may be helpful.

Key learning points

- In a child with a VP shunt, careful history and examination to ensure good shunt function is important prior to anaesthesia.
- If a caudal or lumbar epidural block is used, slow injection will prevent rise in ICP.
- To prolong the duration of single-injection caudal blocks, clonidine, ketamine or opioids may be very effective.
- Continuous epidural analgesia for 48 hours is the technique of choice for intermediate and complex hypospadias corrections.

Further reading

COOK, B. and DOYLE, E. (1996). The use of additives to local anaesthetic solutions for caudal epidural blockade. *Paed. Anaesth.*, **6**, 353–9.
LUMB, A. B. and CARLI, F. (1989). Respiratory arrest after a caudal injection of bupivacaine. *Anaesthesia*, **44**, 324–5.
WILDSMITH, J. A. W. (1986). Extradural blockade and intracranial pressure. *Br. J. Anaesth.*, **58**, 579.

Case 28

A 12-day-old baby born at 30 weeks presents for laparotomy for necrotizing enterocolitis (NEC).

Questions

1. What is necrotizing enterocolitis? List the risk factors and the indications for surgery.
2. Discuss the important points of preoperative preparation.

3. Describe your anaesthetic plan and summarize the major perioperative problems you anticipate.

Answers

1. Necrotizing enterocolitis (NEC) is an acute abdominal condition characterized by gut wall necrosis and intramural air ('pneumatosis intestinalis'). The overall incidence of NEC is 0.3–2.4 per 1000 live births, and it principally affects premature babies who have survived the immediate neonatal period (i.e. those between 7 and 14 days of age). Only about 10 per cent of cases occur in full-term babies, usually at a younger postnatal age (i.e. within 4 days of birth). NEC is most often sporadic, but occasionally outbreaks occur (see Stoll, 1994; Foglia, 1995). The signs and symptoms associated with NEC are given in Table 28.1.

The pathophysiology is multifactorial but not fully understood. Gut ischaemia, formula feeds (but not breast milk), bowel immaturity, and bacterial infection are all implicated (see Albanese and Rowe, 1995; Stoll, 1995; Neu, 1996).

Many risk factors for NEC have been suggested, including:

a. Premature birth and low birth weight
b. Birth asphyxia or respiratory distress
c. Polycythaemia
d. Catheterization of the umbilical vessels
e. Congenital heart disease
f. Blood or exchange transfusion

Table 28.1 Signs and symptoms associated with necrotizing enterocolitis (see Kanto *et al.*, 1994)

Gastrointestinal	Systemic
Abdominal distension	Lethargy
Abdominal tenderness	Apnoea/respiratory distress
Feeding intolerance	Temperature instability
Delayed gastric emptying	'Not right'
Vomiting	Acidosis (metabolic and/or respiratory)
Occult/gross blood in stool	Poor perfusion/shock
Change in stool pattern/diarrhoea	Disseminated intravascular coagulopathy
Abdominal mass	Positive blood cultures
Erythema of abdominal wall	

g. Early and rapid feeding
h. Maternal abuse of cocaine
i. Certain medications (e.g. vitamin E, theophylline and indomethacin)
j. Prolonged rupture of the membranes or chorioamnionitis
k. Antecedent bowel perforation.

However, other authors have failed to identify risk factors in preterm babies other than the prematurity itself (see Foglia, 1994; Kosloske, 1994; Rescorla, 1995). In contrast, mature babies seem to have definite associated features (e.g. congenital heart disease, hypoxia, exchange transfusion). Possibly the disease in premature babies is primarily due to gut immaturity, but requires a specific insult in those born near term (see Stoll, 1994).

The severity of the condition is classified according to the scheme in Table 28.2. The early features of NEC are difficult to differentiate from sepsis, and the initial treatment is supportive. Up to half of babies with NEC have laparotomies, usually those with stages IIIa or b. The indications for surgery are given in Table 28.3 (see also Rescorla, 1995).

2. Babies needing a laparotomy for NEC are very ill and can deteriorate rapidly. Systemic signs suggesting severe sepsis often predominate. The important points of preoperative assessment and preparation are as follows (Kanto *et al.*, 1994; Foglia, 1995).

Identification of conditions associated with prematurity
NEC most commonly affects babies born prematurely. The complications of premature birth include respiratory distress, intraventricular haemorrhage, anaemia, and difficult venous access. These babies may also have congenital anomalies which of themselves are associated with premature birth (e.g. congenital heart disease or tracheo-oesophageal fistula).

Respiratory system
Apnoea is a frequent and often presenting symptom. Respiratory function may be further impaired by the distended abdomen. Initially there will be a combined metabolic and respiratory acidosis, but as the baby becomes sicker the metabolic component dominates because of intestinal ischaemia or poor peripheral perfusion. Babies with NEC usually need ventilatory support with intubation of the trachea and positive pressure ventilation of the lungs. An excessively high inspired concentration of oxygen

Table 28.2 Modified Bell staging criteria for necrotizing enterocolitis

Stage	Classification	Systemic signs	Intestinal signs	Radiological signs
Ia	Suspected NEC	Temperature instability, apnoea, bradycardia, lethargy	Increased gastric aspirates, mid-abdominal distension, vomiting, guaiac-positive stool	Normal/intestinal dilatation, mild ileus
Ib	Suspected NEC	As above	Bright red blood per rectum	As above
IIa	Proven NEC, mildly ill	As above	As above plus absent bowel sounds, with or without abdominal tenderness	Intestinal dilatation, ileus, pneumatosis intestinalis
IIb	Proven NEC, moderately ill	As above, plus mild metabolic acidosis and mild thrombocytopenia	As above plus absent bowel sounds, definite abdominal tenderness with or without abdominal cellulitis or right lower quadrant mass	As IIa plus portal vein gas, with or without ascites
IIIa	Advanced NEC, severely ill, bowel intact	Same as IIb, plus hypotension, bradycardia, severe apnoea, respiratory and metabolic acidosis, disseminated intravascular coagulation and neutropenia	As above, plus signs of generalized peritonitis, marked tenderness and abdominal distension	As IIb plus definite ascites
IIIb	As above, bowel perforated	Same as IIIa	Same as IIIa	As IIb plus pneumoperitoneum

Table 28.3 Indications for operation (see Ricketts, 1994)

Absolute indications
- pneumoperitoneum
- intestinal gangrene (positive results of paracentesis)

Relative indications
- clinical deterioration (metabolic acidosis; ventilatory failure; oliguria; hypovolaemia; thrombocytopenia; leucopenia; leucocytosis)
- portal vein gas
- erythema of abdominal wall
- fixed abdominal mass
- persistently dilated loop

Non-indications
- severe gastrointestinal haemorrhage
- abdominal tenderness
- intestinal obstruction
- gasless abdomen with ascites

should be avoided to reduce the risk of retinopathy of pre-maturity, but adequate oxygen delivery must be ensured. The aim is a P_aO_2 of 6.7–9.1 kPa, and an attempt should be made to correct any acidosis with a combination of positive pressure ventilation, fluid resuscitation and inotropic support (see below).

Circulatory system and fluid balance

NEC is often associated with large shifts of fluid into the 'third space' and signs of septic shock. Hypovolaemia must be corrected using a combination of colloid (e.g. albumen 4.5%) and crystalloid (e.g. 0.9% saline), maintenance fluids should be increased by up to 150 per cent, and gastric aspirates replaced with adequate amounts of water and electrolytes. These babies often require large volumes of fluid, and adequate venous access must be ensured. To assess haemodynamic variables, the anaesthetist will probably need to monitor central venous pressure and intra-arterial blood pressure. The normal systolic pressure in a new-born ranges from about 45 mmHg in those weighing 1 kg to about 65 mmHg in those of 3 kg. The urine output should be 1.5–2 ml/kg per hour.

Electrolytes should be measured every 8–12 hours because changes are unpredictable, and supplements should then be pre-scribed according to plasma concentrations. Particular care must be taken with potassium; hyperkalaemia can result from bowel necrosis or impaired renal function.

Oxygen delivery should be optimized by ensuring an adequate intravascular volume and then treating poor perfusion or hypotension with inotropes (e.g. dopamine 3–15 μg/kg per minute; dobutamine 5–15 μg/kg per minute). Excessive α effects can further compromise gut perfusion.

Haematological system

Moderate to severe NEC is associated with thrombocytopenia and disseminated intravascular coagulation. The aim should be a platelet count of at least 50×10^9/l, and deficient clotting factors should be replaced before surgery. One unit of platelet concentrate per 5 kg body weight should increase the platelet count by 50×10^9/l; 10–15 ml/kg of fresh frozen plasma supplies all clotting factors in limited quantity; and one unit of cryoprecipitate per 5 kg body weight will increase the fibrinogen concentration by 0.75 g/l (see Gordon et al., 1995).

The haemoglobin concentration should be checked and any anaemia corrected, aiming for a haematocrit of 35–40 per cent. Anaemia is common in premature babies, and may be worsened by bleeding from the bowel. Conversely, significant loss of fluid from the intravascular space in NEC may produce haemoconcentration. Laparotomy is associated with large blood losses, so cross-matched blood should be requested before surgery.

Glucose

The glucose may be normal, high or low, and should be measured regularly. Babies are particularly likely to become hypoglycaemic, because they have limited glycogen stores. Hypoglycaemia (i.e. a plasma glucose concentration < 2.2 mmol/l) should be treated promptly with 5 ml/kg of glucose 10%.

Sepsis

Blood cultures are positive in 30–35 per cent of babies, and most commonly grow *Klebsiella pneumoniae* or *Escherichia coli* (see Albanese and Rowe, 1995). It is not known if these are the pathogens causing NEC or simply opportunistic bacteria.

Blood should be taken for culture and broad-spectrum antibiotics prescribed to cover those bacteria commonly associated with NEC. The known prevalence of organisms and the patterns of resistance on the neonatal intensive care unit should also be taken into account.

Temperature regulation

Babies with NEC have impaired regulation of temperature and are particularly prone to hypothermia. Core and peripheral temperatures should be monitored and these babies nursed within an incubator or beneath a radiant heater.

Gastric stasis

NEC produces an ileus. To reduce the risk of pulmonary aspiration of gastric contents at the induction of anaesthesia, the anaesthetist should decompress the stomach preoperatively with a gastric tube.

3. Babies having surgery for NEC should be managed in a centre with adequate facilities for the sickest preterm babies. They should be cared for only by anaesthetists and surgeons with adequate training and continuing clinical experience. The anaesthetic plan should take account of the basic principles of anaesthesia for any preterm baby (i.e. appropriate equipment, trained assistance, consideration of age-related physiology and pharmacology etc.) and the specific problems in NEC. These babies often have a stormy intraoperative course, and it is advisable to have a second anaesthetist to help.

   Most babies will be intubated, mechanically ventilated and receiving intravenous fluids as part of their preoperative resuscitation. In those not intubated, precautions must be taken to reduce the risk of aspiration of gastric contents during the induction of anaesthesia (i.e. aspiration of the gastric tube and use of a rapid sequence induction with pre-oxygenation, cricoid pressure and suxamethonium). The choices of induction agent and non-depolarizing muscle relaxant are not important, because the baby will almost certainly be ventilated postoperatively. The dose of induction agent should be reduced in unstable babies; thiopentone 2 mg/kg is appropriate. Alternatively, fentanyl 5–10 μg/kg may be given.

   Anaesthesia can be maintained with a low inspired concentration of a volatile agent (e.g. 0.5% isoflurane) in oxygen-enriched air. Nitrous oxide is contraindicated because of the presence of air within the wall of the bowel. The inspired oxygen concentration should be the minimum to maintain adequate oxygen saturation to reduce the risks of retinopathy of prematurity. If an arterial cannula has been inserted, the arterial partial pressure of oxygen and carbon dioxide can be checked. A transcutaneous oxygen probe is unreliable because the probe is easily dislodged during surgery. Adequate anaesthesia (e.g. fentanyl 10–100 μg/kg in divided doses) will reduce the stress of surgery. The elimination of fentanyl may be delayed because of decreased hepatic blood flow secondary to raised intra-abdominal pressure postoperatively. Epidural analgesia is not appropriate because of the associated coagulopathy. In addition, the baby will be ventilated mechanically for several days after surgery, and sedatives (usually morphine) will be given. The risk of epidural infection is increased in NEC due to bacteraemia seeding onto the epidural catheter.

In addition to those problems seen preoperatively (e.g. hypotension, a coagulopathy, hypoglycaemia), the following difficulties can be expected during surgery.

Massive fluid losses

Large fluid losses should be anticipated (e.g. from bleeding, evaporation and oedema). Adequate venous access must be available (two relatively large cannulae), and the anaesthetist must be prepared to infuse relatively large volumes of fluid (i.e. blood and plasma) rapidly. Because of the large fluid loss and the potential for cardiovascular instability (see below), it is useful to monitor the central venous and intra-arterial pressures.

A coagulopathy is common, and it may be worth using fresh frozen plasma to maintain normovolaemia from the outset in very sick babies.

Spontaneous liver haemorrhage is common during surgery, particularly in those babies needing the greatest volume of fluid resuscitation preoperatively. Excessive fluid may cause expansion of the liver capsule and predispose to bleeding. Babies with liver haemorrhage have a huge increase in perioperative mortality compared to those without (87 per cent compared to 12 per cent).

Citrate toxicity

Hypotension is common, and may result from inadequate fluid resuscitation, massive haemorrhage, the 'sepsis syndrome' (see above), or citrate toxicity.

Citrate binds to ionized calcium. This rarely causes a problem in older children and adults because citrate is metabolized rapidly in the liver, but babies, particularly those who are very ill, have a limited capacity for metabolism of citrate. Hypocalcaemia may become clinically apparent (with hypotension and a tachycardia) during transfusion of blood products containing citrate. Fresh frozen plasma given in excess of 1–2.5 ml/kg per minute may produce significant hypocalcaemia. Ionized calcium should be measured during surgery and deficiencies replaced as 10% calcium chloride 0.1 ml/kg slowly into a central vein.

Hypothermia

NEC and anaesthesia significantly impair temperature regulation. In addition, a baby loses relatively more heat than an adult during surgery because of a larger surface area : weight ratio, reduced insulation of the body core, smaller radii of curvature of body surfaces (increases radiation), greater permeability of the skin to water (see Darnall, 1987), and a large head. They will lose a huge amount of heat from evaporation from the abdominal cavity and bowels during laparotomy, and can easily become hypothermic during the infusion of large volumes of fluids or from washing out the abdominal cavity.

All fluids infused (other than maintenance fluids) or used for abdominal washouts should be warmed to 37 °C. Evaporative heat losses can be reduced by covering some of the abdominal contents with warmed saline soaks or polythene, and by draping the baby with a waterproof material to prevent pooling of fluid around the baby.

Other precautions to reduce heat loss include increasing the ambient temperature and humidity (25°C and 50 per cent relative humidity), excluding draughts, active heating and humidification of inspired gases, using an overhead radiant heater whenever the baby is exposed, and reducing conductive losses to the operating table with a warming blanket.

The most common postoperative complications are sepsis (particularly in babies with very low birth weight), intestinal strictures and short bowel syndrome, or multi-organ failure. Others include complications from central venous cannulation, parenteral nutrition, or coexistent medical problems (e.g. respiratory or congenital heart disease).

Mortality in babies needing surgery for NEC is about 40 per cent. A gestational age less than 27 weeks and weight below 1000 g at birth is associated with a particularly poor outcome. Death usually results from:

a. Refractory shock
b. Disseminated intravascular coagulation
c. Multiple organ failure
d. Intestinal perforation and sepsis

e. Extensive bowel necrosis
f. Short bowel syndrome (see Stoll, 1994).

Key learning points

- NEC is a high risk, multifactorial cause of acute abdomen in neonates.
- Stabilization prior to surgery needs to be meticulous and vigorous.
- Invasive monitoring is recommended.
- Epidural analgesia is relatively contraindicated by coagulopathy and bacteraemia.

Further reading

ALBANESE, C. T. and ROWE, M. (1995). Necrotizing enterocolitis. *Sem. Ped. Surg.*, **4**, 200–206.

DARNALL, R. A. (1987). The thermophysiology of the newborn infant. *Med. Inst.*, **21**, 16–22.

FOGLIA, R. P. (1995). Necrotizing enterocolitis. *Curr. Prob. Surg.*, **32**, 759–823.

GORDON, J. B., BERNSTEIN, M. I. and ROGERS, M. C. (1995). Hematologic disorders in the pediatric intensive care unit. In: *Handbook of Pediatric Intensive Care*, 2nd edn (M. C. Rogers and M. A. Helfaer, eds), Ch. 23, pp. 657–87. Williams & Wilkins.

KANTO, W. P., HUNTER, J. E., STOLL, B. J. *et al.* (1994). Recognition and medical management of necrotizing enterocolitis. *Clin. Perinatol.*, **21**, 335–46.

KOSLOSKE, A. M. (1994). Epidemiology of necrotizing enterocolitis. *Acta Paed.* (Suppl.), **396**, 2–7.

NEU, J. (1996). Necrotizing enterocolitis. *Ped. Clin. North Am.*, **43**, 409–32.

RESCORLA, F. J. (1995). Surgical management of pediatric necrotizing enterocolitis. *Curr. Opin. Ped.*, **7**, 335–41.

RICKETTS, R. R. (1994). Surgical treatment of necrotizing enterocolitis and the short bowel syndrome. *Clin. Perinatol.*, **21**, 365–87.

STOLL, B. J. (1994). Epidemiology of necrotizing enterocolitis. *Clin. Perinatol.*, **21**, 205–18.

Case 29

A 5-week-old baby boy presents with a 3-day history of projectile vomiting. A diagnosis of hypertrophy of the pylorus has been made on ultrasound examination, and the surgeons have listed him for a pyloromyotomy. The baby is adequately resuscitated and has normal electrolytes. He has an intravenous infusion and nasogastric tube. On preoperative assessment, you note he has profound micrognathia.

Questions

1. Describe the airway abnormalities and methods of management of the Pierre–Robin syndrome.
2. List the clinical associations.
3. How will you manage the airway during anaesthesia?

Answers

1. Pierre–Robin syndrome consists of micrognathia (hypoplasia of the mandible), pseudo-macroglossia and glossoptosis (the posterior tongue is displaced posteriorly and downwards against the prevertebral tissues of the pharynx). These abnormalities can significantly obstruct the airway, causing hypercarbia, difficulty in feeding and failure to thrive. The airway is usually clearer with the baby lying prone or laterally, but it can deteriorate during feeding or in the prone position. Techniques used to improve the airway include (see Buchman, 1996):

   a. Nursing the baby prone to allow the tongue to fall forward – an adapted bed is available to maintain this position.
   b. Inserting a nasopharyngeal airway.
   c. Suturing the tongue to the lip to pull the tongue away from the posterior pharyngeal wall.

   If significant airway obstruction persists despite these techniques, a tracheostomy may be indicated. The airway tends to improve as the mandible grows with age.
2. Pierre–Robin syndrome is associated with cleft palate in 90 per cent and with other anomalies in about 50 per cent of affected babies. The most frequent associations are musculoskeletal, cardiac or other cranio-facial malformations. Psychomotor retardation occurs in about a quarter of affected babies. Mortality is increased in babies with more severe symptoms or associated congenital abnormalities, and in those born prematurely.
3. This baby has two serious problems for anaesthesia: a difficult airway and the potential risks of a full stomach. Preventing aspiration by using a rapid sequence induction may produce

a disastrous loss of the airway and is contraindicated. The risk of aspiration during anaesthesia can be reduced by carefully aspirating stomach contents through the nasogastric tube. The anaesthetist should do this with the baby in several positions. Some paediatric anaesthetists currently do not use a rapid sequence induction even in normal babies with pyloric stenosis.

Several techniques for intubating the trachea in babies with Pierre–Robin syndrome have been described (see below). It is essential that the anaesthetist has a clear plan of management and is adequately prepared, because it is impossible to fully assess this baby's airway before surgery. The following are necessary:

a. Trained personnel, including: an experienced paediatric fibre-optic laryngoscopist; an additional experienced anaesthetist; trained assistance and an experienced paediatric ear, nose and throat surgeon.

b. A range of equipment that should be obtained and prepared in advance (Table 29.1), including equipment for needle cricothyroidotomy and oxygen insufflation (Table 29.2).

Secretions that may further compromise the airway during induction of anaesthesia can be reduced with an antisialogue administered intravenously (glycopyrrolate 10 μg/kg or atropine 20 μg/kg). Minimal monitoring (oximetry and electrocardiograph) should be established before inducing anaesthesia, and capnography and non-invasive blood pressure monitoring should be available.

Table 29.1 Equipment for managing a difficult airway in a baby

Tracheal and pharyngeal suction catheters
Magill's forceps
Face pieces
Oropharyngeal and nasopharyngeal airways
Laryngeal mask airway size 1
Tracheal tubes sizes 2.0–3.5
Malleable tracheal tube introducers
Range of neonatal laryngoscope blades, e.g. Miller, Robertshaw, Bullard
Neonatal and adult fibre-optic laryngoscopes, appropriately sized Seldinger wires and suction tubing
Equipment for cricothyroid puncture and oxygen insufflation (see Table 29.2)
Light wand (optional)
Anterior commissure laryngoscope with optical stylette (optional)

Table 29.2 Needle cricothyroidotomy and oxygen insufflation (see Advanced Life Support Group, 1997)

Equipment required
Oxygen tubing connected at one end to 15-l/min oxygen outlet from the wall and to a three-way tap at the other; 19G cannula; 5-ml syringe

Technique of cricothyroidotomy
The baby's head is gently extended over a roll. The cricothyroid membrane is identified and the skin cleaned with antiseptic solution. The needle and cannula (with the syringe attached) are advanced at an angle of 45° caudally through the skin and cricothyroid membrane, aspirating continuously The trachea is identified when air is aspirated. The cannula is then advanced over the needle, which is withdrawn. The position of the tip of the cannula is reconfirmed by aspirating air again. The hub of the cannula is then attached to the three-way tap open in all directions.

Technique of oxygen insufflation
The oxygen flow meter is adjusted to 1 l/min. The three-way tap is occluded with the thumb for 1 s, and movement of the chest assessed. Passive exhalation is permitted by removing the thumb for 4 s. If chest wall movement is inadequate, oxygen flow is increased by increments of 1 l/min.

Whatever technique is used for the induction of anaesthesia and intubation of the trachea, it is essential that the baby is positioned correctly. His head can be maintained in a more neutral position by placing a roll under the shoulders to compensate for the relatively large occiput.

The airway can be difficult to maintain with the baby supine, even if awake, and deteriorates after the induction of anaesthesia. It is often improved by a nasal airway. The length of the airway is estimated by measuring from the nares to the tragus. It needs to be long enough to overcome the obstruction caused by the back of the tongue, but not so long that its tip passes into the oesophagus. The patency of the airway may be further improved by applying continuous positive airway pressure.

The laryngeal mask airway (LMA) often provides an excellent airway in babies with the Pierre–Robin syndrome. The LMA is usually inserted after the induction of anaesthesia, but can be introduced after topical anaesthesia of the oropharynx in awake babies. The LMA can be used to deliver anaesthetic gases during spontaneous and intermittent positive pressure ventilation, and as a conduit to facilitate other techniques of tracheal intubation. Muscle relaxants should be considered before intubation only if positive pressure ventilation through the nasopharyngeal or LM airway is easy.

Intubation of the trachea is not essential in this baby, but it will provide a more secure airway and reduce the risk of aspirating gastric contents during manipulation of the bowel. The trachea can be intubated with the baby awake or anaesthetized. Intubation using conventional techniques of laryngoscopy in awake babies is difficult and traumatic, and is associated with an increased incidence of hypoxia. Advanced techniques of tracheal intubation have been reported in awake babies with Pierre–Robin syndrome after topical anaesthesia of the airway. Lignocaine can be given by nebulizer (total dose of 3 mg/kg).

Several techniques and adjuncts can be used to intubate the trachea.

Conventional laryngoscopy

Intubation using a conventional straight-bladed laryngoscope may be successful. Certain manoeuvres may help improve the view of the larynx – e.g. inserting the 'scope from the extreme right- or left-hand corner of the mouth, cricoid pressure, anterior traction on the tongue etc. (see Bosenberg, 1996). Bougies or stiffening tubes with flexible introducers may permit intubation despite a poor view of the larynx.

Other designs of laryngoscope may be helpful. The Bullard 'scope has been used to obtain a satisfactory view of the larynx in a baby with Pierre–Robin syndrome whose glottis could not be visualized with standard blades. The Bullard 'scope has an anatomically-shaped rigid blade with a bend of 90° over which a tracheal tube or bougie can be passed, and a light source and image bundle to give a view of the tip (see Bosenberg, 1996; Reynolds, 1996). It can be introduced with minimal mouth opening. The anterior commissure laryngoscope used by ear, nose and throat surgeons is an alternative that may facilitate tracheal intubation (see Reynolds, 1996).

Insertion of tracheal tube 'blindly'

Passing a tube blindly through the LMA has been described, but is probably not recommended because in more than half of babies and children the epiglottis will either impinge onto the grille of the LMA or be folded downwards. The tracheal tube may then impinge on the vallecula and cause trauma. Alternatively, the larynx can assessed with a fibrescope passed through the LMA first and the tube passed 'blindly' only if the view is satisfactory.

Fibre-optic laryngoscopy

Seldinger wire technique. A flexible guide wire can be inserted through the suction port of the adult fibre-optic bronchoscope (external diameter 3.5 mm) and subsequently used as a guide for a tracheal tube. The adult 'scope is easier to use and has a suction port to aspirate secretions or insufflate oxygen. The 'scope is introduced through a modification of a face mask, the nose or, more commonly, an LMA (Figure 29.1). The baby may be awake, but is usually anaesthetized. Unless the lungs can be ventilated easily, the baby should breathe spontaneously. Once viewed, the larynx is sprayed with lignocaine (maximum dose 3 mg/kg) to reduce coughing and laryngospasm and after 1 minute the wire is advanced through the vocal cords. In larger babies and children the fibrescope can also be advanced into the trachea. The 'scope is removed carefully without displacing the wire, and the wire then acts to guide the tracheal tube. The discrepancy between the tracheal tube and the wire may be reduced by first passing either a urethral catheter or dilator or

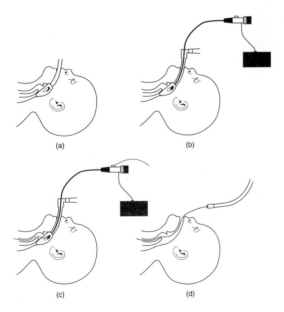

(a)

(b)

(c)

(d)

Figure 1 (a) insertion of LMA; **(b)** visualizing the LMA grille and the glottis with the fibrescope; **(c)** insertion of the guide wire into the trachea through the suction port of the fibrescope **(d)** insertion of the tracheal tube over the guide wire

an angiography catheter over the wire. This stiffens the guide and may reduce the risk of the tube impinging on the larynx. The risk is probably also reduced by using a flexible, spirally reinforced tube.

The passage of the tube into the trachea can also be observed using the above technique by inserting the 'scope through the other nostril (see Reynolds, 1996). Alternatively, the Seldinger wire can be passed into the trachea under direct vision but not through the suction port. This obviates the need to remove the fibrescope and allows the anaesthetist to observe the insertion of the tracheal tube through the vocal cords.

'Rail-roading' a tracheal tube over a 2.2- or 1.8-mm external diameter fibrescope. The neonatal fibrescope has an external diameter of 2.2 mm, allowing a tracheal tube as small as 2.5 mm to be loaded onto it. The 'ultrathin' fibrescope with an external diameter of 1.8 mm has also been used to facilitate tracheal intubation in babies with difficult airways. The trachea can be cannulated with the 'scope and the tube passed over it in babies who are awake or anaesthetized. This technique allows the position of the tracheal tube to be confirmed at the initial laryngoscopy, and there is less potential to decannulate the trachea during the procedure compared with the Seldinger wire technique. However, the fine 'scopes have no suction port, are more difficult to use, and are associated with a relatively high incidence of failed or difficult orotracheal intubations in older babies. These difficulties may be explained by the higher position of the larynx in babies, requiring a more acute curve to the tracheal tube, and by using relatively large tubes over small diameter 'scopes'.

If it is difficult to advance the tracheal tube, simple manoeuvres such as flexing the neck, using a jaw thrust, pressing backwards on the larynx, rotating the tube 90° clockwise or anticlockwise, or using reinforced tubes can help.

Light-wand technique
A flexible light wand can be used to facilitate intubation (see Bosenberg, 1996; Reynolds, 1996), using equipment specifically designed for babies. A fibre-optic laryngoscope can be utilized as a light wand, and this technique has been described in a baby with Pierre–Robin syndrome.

Retrograde tracheal cannulation
Retrograde tracheal cannulation has been described using an 18G cannula and a 25G catheter in a baby with Goldenhar syndrome,

but the technique is difficult and has serious potential complications (surgical emphysema, bleeding, laryngospasm and airway oedema), and the landmarks are ill defined (see Bosenberg, 1996). The tracheal tube can be difficult to pass through the larynx.

Key learning points

- Pierre–Robin syndrome is often associated with cleft palate and other anomalies.
- A strategy for difficult intubation with options should be carefully planned.
- Techniques based upon the LMA have proven to be extremely useful in such cases.

Further reading

BOSENBERG, A. (1996). Difficult intubation in neonates and small infants. In: *Handbook of Neonatal Anaesthesia* (D. G. Hughes, S. J. Mather and A. R. Wolf, eds), Ch. 12, pp. 298–320. W. B. Saunders.
BUCHMAN, S. (1996). Clinical problems of the difficult airway in craniofacial surgery. In: *Atlas of the Difficult Airway*, 2nd edn (M. L. Norton, ed.), Ch. 15, pp. 226–44. Mosby.
REYNOLDS, P. (1996). Pediatric difficult airways. In: *Atlas of the Difficult Airway*, 2nd edn (M. L. Norton, ed.), Ch. 16, pp. 245–66. Mosby.

Case 30

A 2-year-old girl presents to the casualty department with a history of vomiting and inability to retain food or fluids for the past 24 hours. On the chest X-ray, an opacity resembling a coin is visible in the mid-thoracic area. She has no respiratory symptoms, and her parents do not report any choking episodes. She weighs 14 kg.

Questions

1. What should be the initial management of this girl?
2. How would you proceed to anaesthetize her if the coin requires removal?

Answers

1. The history of vomiting and inadequate fluid intake means this patient is potentially dehydrated and may have electrolyte abnormalities. She may be manifesting a degree of intravascular volume depletion with a tachycardia and a cool, pale peripheral circulation and sluggish capillary refill. It is also important to ascertain from the parents if there has been blood in the vomit, as this may indicate oesophageal trauma. Initial management should consist of obtaining venous access and taking blood for urea and electrolytes and a full blood count. Intravenous fluids can be commenced at a maintenance rate of 48 ml/h, although any degree of fluid deficit may need to be replaced in addition to this. If the potassium is low, this should be added to the 0.45% saline and 5% dextrose solution. The child should then be admitted to the ward for observation. The usual progression of events is removal of the coin under general anaesthesia. Very occasionally the coin will pass unaided through the stomach, and then it is usually possible to manage its subsequent passage conservatively.

2. The anaesthetic management commences with a routine preoperative assessment in addition to specific evaluation of volume status. Although in this case there is no history of respiratory embarrassment, the chest and chest X-ray must be examined carefully. There has been one case report of a child treated as asthmatic who was subsequently found to have a coin lodged in the oesophagus and compressing the trachea. It is also important to find out if the girl has had any previous oesophageal trauma or if it is likely that she has swallowed anything else of a more corrosive nature. Oesophagoscopy with a rigid scope carries the risk of potential perforation or damage. This is obviously more likely if the oesophagus has been previously injured, and great care must be taken in these cases.

    Apart from ensuring adequate resuscitation, the specific anaesthetic risk is that of regurgitation or vomiting. In a survey of paediatric anaesthetists in the United States, rapid sequence induction was the preferred technique for the removal of foreign bodies in the gastrointestinal tract. This was in contrast to the preferred technique of inhalational induction with spontaneous respiration for foreign body in the airway.

This would also be the case in the UK, and thus the girl should undergo a rapid-sequence induction using thiopentone 5–7 mg/kg and suxamethonium 1–3 mg/kg. A size 4.5 plain oral endotracheal tube is appropriate, and cricoid pressure should be applied until the airway is secured. A rigid oesophagoscope is used to visualize the coin and facilitate its removal with long forceps. It is imperative that the child is adequately anaesthetized and does not cough during the procedure, as this may incur the risk of oesophageal damage. Therefore a non-depolarizing muscle relaxant such as atracurium, vecuronium or mivacurium is often required after the suxamethonium has worn off. It is necessary to wait the appropriate length of time prior to reversal of the neuromuscular blockade after the successful removal of the coin. Postoperatively the child should continue to receive intravenous fluids until drinking comfortably, and she should be observed for a signs indicating oesophageal trauma or mediastinitis.

Key learning points

- Careful preoperative assessment of the child's state of hydration and the coin position is essential.
- Rapid sequence induction and subsequent use of non-depolarizing relaxants is recommended.

Further reading

KAIN, Z. N., O'CONNOR, T. Z. and BERDE, C. B. (1994). Management of tracheobronchial and esophageal foreign bodies in children: a survey study. *J. Clin. Anesth.*, **6(1)**, 28–32.

JONA, J. .Z., GLICKLICH, M. and COHEN, R. D. (1998). The contraindications for blind oesophageal bouginage for caustic ingestion in children. *J. Ped. Surg.*, **23(4)**, 328–30.

Case 31

A 13-month-old girl presents for an inguinal hernia repair. She had an upper respiratory tract infection 3 weeks ago, but is otherwise well with no significant past medical history. She weighs

12 kg and is very chubby. You can find no veins, and choose an inhalational induction of anaesthesia with sevoflurane in oxygen and nitrous oxide and change to isoflurane when anaesthesia is considered to be sufficiently deep. On attempting to insert a number 2 laryngeal mask airway (LMA) before cannulating a vein, the child develops marked stridor and partial airway obstruction.

Questions

1. What is the cause of stridor in this girl? Discuss the mechanism of airway obstruction.
2. Discuss the plan of management.
3. List the short-term complications.

Answers

1. Stridor is most likely caused by the early stages of laryngo-spasm.

   The precise pathophysiology of laryngospasm is unclear but seems to involve prolonged adduction of the true vocal cords, sometimes with simultaneous adduction of the false cords. The false cords and supraglottic structures may contribute to airway obstruction (see Roy and Lerman, 1988); during laryngospasm the thyrohyoid muscles shorten and the supra-glottic tissues become rounded and redundant. As the pressure gradient increases during attempted inspiration these tissues are drawn together and down into the laryngeal inlet, worsening obstruction. Inspiration may also cause a Venturi effect, pulling the cords closer together and further narrowing the laryngeal opening (see Landsman, 1997). Passive relaxation of the abductors may contribute to partial closure of the glottis.

   Spasm is mediated by the superior laryngeal nerve in response to a variety of stimuli, e.g. irritating inhalational anaesthetic agents, secretions, manipulation of the airway or stimulation of visceral nerves in the chest, abdomen and pelvis. The duration of glottic closure exceeds the duration of the stimulus that caused it. The incidence is increased by upper respiratory tract infections (see Landsman, 1997).

Adductor muscle activity is increased by hypocapnia or lung deflation and reduced by hypercapnia, severe hypoxia (< 50 mmHg) and inflation of the lungs. These experimental observations support the clinical impression that laryngospasm is broken by profound hypoxia, hypercarbia or shock (Roy and Lerman, 1988; Landsman, 1997).

2. In the initial management of laryngospasm, the stimulus (i.e. the LMA and irritant volatile anaesthetic agent) should be removed, 100 per cent oxygen given and an attempt made to deepen the level of anaesthesia. Bradycardia is a significant response to severe or prolonged hypoxia in children, and it is essential to monitor the electrocardiogram and oxygen saturation.

Oxygenation may be adequate if additional continuous positive airway pressure is given through a closely fitting face-mask. If inadequate oxygenation persists, the next step would be to try to ventilate the lungs with oxygen. This may be possible if the laryngospasm is incomplete or the obstruction is due to passive relaxation of the laryngeal muscles. In complete airway obstruction, positive airway pressure may simply distend the pyriform fossae on either side of the larynx and force the aryteno-epiglottic folds even closer together. It may be possible to improve the airway by opening the laryngeal aperture with a jaw thrust; the force applied is transmitted through ligaments and muscles to unfold the supraglottic structures, pulling the paraglottis away from the false cords (Roy and Lerman, 1988; Landsman, 1997). If these techniques fail to improve or maintain adequate oxygenation, the laryngospasm must be broken by either deepening the depth of anaesthesia or giving a muscle relaxant.

Increasing the depth of anaesthesia

Anaesthesia can be deepened with a small dose of induction agent if intravenous access is easily obtained (see below) or, if the airway is only partially obstructed, by carefully increasing the inspired concentration of a non-irritant volatile agent. Sevoflurane is the agent of choice because it is relatively non-irritant to the airways and is associated with stable cardiac rhythms. Halothane is less suitable because it depresses cardiac automaticity and conduction, facilitating re-entrant and nodal arrhythmias (e.g. ventricular tachycardia). These rhythms are more likely in hypoxia or if intrinsic catecholamine concentrations are raised.

Muscle relaxants

Suxamethonium works rapidly, and can be given by several routes.

Intravenous injection. It may be possible to cannulate a vein. In the absence of obvious veins in the backs of the hands, good places to look are the ankle (the long saphenous vein) and the neck (external jugular vein). The landmark for the long saphenous at the ankle is half a finger-breadth in babies (one finger-breadth in small children) superior and anterior to the medial malleolus. The vein can often be cannulated quickly with a 'blind' technique if the vessel can neither be seen nor palpated. The external jugular · can often be found, even in fat babies. The baby's head should be turned away from the site of cannulation with the child 15–30° head down. The vein is seen as it passes over the sternomastoid muscle. There may also be suitable veins over the abdomen and chest or in the scalp.

If intravenous access is obtained quickly, suxamethonium can be injected to relax the vocal cords and permit positive pressure ventilation of the lungs. Laryngospasm may be broken in adults with even small doses of suxamethonium (0.1 mg/kg), allowing the depth of anaesthesia to be deepened rapidly before the muscle relaxation has resolved. A larger dose of suxamethonium may be chosen to facilitate intubation of the trachea and secure the airway. However, stridor associated with extubation is also common, and the anaesthetist may opt to continue inhalational anaesthesia through an LMA or facemask, ensuring an adequate depth of anaesthesia throughout. If the anaesthetist elects to intubate the trachea, the risk of laryngospasm at extubation may be reduced if the cords are sprayed with lignocaine. It is uncertain whether intravenous lignocaine before extubation is effective.

Intramuscular or intralingual injection of suxamethonium. Suxamethonium can be injected into muscle (e.g. into the quadriceps femoris or deltoid) or the tongue. Apnoea in children given suxamethonium 1 mg/kg occurs in a mean of 75 s with intralingual and 35 s with intravenous injection. The effects are significantly delayed if injected into skeletal muscle: 2 mg/kg intramuscularly (deltoid or quadriceps femoris) produces apnoea after a mean of 3.5 min. There is no clinically significant difference in the mean time to reduction of twitch height to 10 per cent of control between the tongue and the quadriceps femoris (295 ± 43 s for quadriceps femoris compared with 265 ± 62.5 s for the intralingual route when given 3 mg/kg). However, massage of the tongue decreases the time to 133 ± 12 s. Some authors recommend suxamethonium 4 mg/kg given into the deltoid muscle to treat laryngospasm. Although the mean maximum reduction in twitch height measured in the thumb occurs at just less than 4 minutes, the intrinsic muscles of the larynx seem very sensitive to suxamethonium and control of the airway improves much more rapidly. Satisfactory conditions for intubation of the trachea will take a while longer.

Intramuscular suxamethonium, compared with intravenous or intralingual, is associated with few or no cardiac arrhythmias. Intralingual suxamethonium is associated with potentially serious rhythms (e.g. bigeminy, multifocal ventricular ectopics and ventricular tachycardia) in children premedicated with atropine and anaesthetized with halothane. In those not anaesthetized with halothane, atropine 20 μg/kg injected with the suxamethonium has been recommended to reduce the risk of bradycardia caused by hypoxia or suxamethonium (Roy and Lerman, 1988).

Intraosseous injection. Access to the circulation in children younger than 6 years can be obtained through an intraosseous needle if intravenous cannulation is not possible or takes too long. The needle is usually inserted through the anterior surface of the tibia 2–3 cm below the tibial tuberosity. Alternative sites are the medial surface of the tibia 3 cm above the medial malleolus, and the distal femur 3 cm above the lateral condyle. All drugs used in cardiopulmonary resuscitation and a variety of others including suxamethonium, thiopentone and atropine can be injected. The onset of action of drugs is almost as fast as intravenous injection. However, the technique takes a couple of minutes and control of the airway is probably best obtained rapidly by giving suxamethonium into the tongue as described above. If the clinical situation deteriorates despite this, intraosseous cannulation would be indicated.

If the situation is extreme (i.e. bradycardia and profound hypoxia) and intramuscular suxamethonium has not had time to work, the anaesthetist should attempt intubation. It may be possible to relax the vocal cords using topical lignocaine (see Roy and Lerman, 1988). Hypoxia and hypercarbia depress adductor muscle activity in the larynx, supporting the clinical observation that the larynx often relaxes during profound hypoxia, finally allowing intermittent positive pressure ventilation with oxygen. However, this does not always occur; in desperation needle cricothyroidotomy and oxygen insufflation may need to be considered.

3. The short-term complications of laryngospasm include gastric dilatation, pulmonary oedema and cardiac arrest.

Gastric dilatation

Gastric dilatation associated with attempted positive pressure ventilation is common. Gastric distension increases the risk of aspirating gastric contents; raises intra-abdominal pressure, decreasing venous return; and splints the diaphragm, impeding ventilation. If marked gastric distension occurs, it is essential that the stomach is decompressed with a large-bore nasogastric tube because it can impede attempts to ventilate the lungs. However, this should only be done if there is obvious swelling of the abdomen; inserting a nasogastric tube is itself a stimulus for laryngospasm.

Pulmonary oedema

Pulmonary oedema can complicate acute airway obstruction in children without other predisposing factors. The aetiology is thought to be multifactorial, and may be explained by the following:

a. Vigorous efforts to breathe against a closed glottis generate very negative intrathoracic pressures. This produces a large pressure gradient across the alveolar–capillary membrane, encouraging fluid to shift from the capillaries into the pulmonary interstitial space, as described by Starling's equation. The high negative pressure also moves blood into the thorax, increasing intrathoracic blood volume and pulmonary blood pressure.
b. Hypoxia may constrict post-capillary sphincters and veins in the pulmonary circulation, increasing capillary pressure and encouraging the movement of fluid into the alveoli. It also depresses myocardial contractility, contributing to the development of pulmonary oedema.
c. Cardiac function is impaired by high negative intrathoracic pressure, and this produces an increase in left atrial and pulmonary blood volumes. Pulmonary capillary pressure then rises, encouraging exudation of fluid into the alveoli.
d. Hypoxia, hypercarbia and stress all increase sympathetic output, which may affect fluid distribution and vascular tone.

The treatment of pulmonary oedema associated with laryngospasm consists of oxygen, continuous positive airway pressure, and positive pressure ventilation if required. Diuretics may be of less value because the pulmonary capillary wedge pressure measured in adults is normal. Frusemide may be useful because it has a secondary action to increase venous capacitance.

Cardiac arrest
Profound hypoxia can cause bradycardia or asystole. Suxamethonium and halothane are associated with serious arrhythmias (e.g. bradycardia, junctional and ventricular arrhythmias). These are potentiated by hypoxia and hypercarbia. Management of cardiac arrest is according to accepted guidelines.

Key learning points

- Laryngospasm is most often due to light anaesthesia, and the incidence is higher in children with upper respiratory tract infection.
- Rapid intervention is essential (remove the stimulus, give oxygen, give CPAP, deepen the level of anaesthesia, give a relaxant).
- If there is no venous access, suxamethonium can be given by the intramuscular, intralingual or intraosseous routes.

Further reading

LANDSMAN, I. S. (1997). Mechanisms and treatment of laryngospasm. *Int. Anesthesiol. Clin.*, **35,** 67–73.
ROY, W. I. and LERMAN, J. (1988). Laryngospasm in paediatric anaesthesia. *Can. J. Anaesth.*, **35,** 93–8.

Case 32

A baby boy with hydrocephalus is listed for insertion of a ventriculo-peritoneal shunt. He is 11 weeks old, and was born at 32 weeks of gestation.

132

Questions

1. What are the causes and clinical signs of hydrocephalus in a baby?
2. Describe your anaesthetic plan and discuss the main problems associated with anaesthesia and surgery.
3. What are your recommendations for postoperative care?

Answers

1. Hydrocephalus is almost always caused by impaired absorption, rather than excessive secretion, of cerebrospinal fluid (CSF). CSF continues to be secreted despite an increase in intracranial pressure. Hydrocephalus can be *communicating* (CSF leaves the ventricular system but absorption by the arachnoid villi is inhibited) or *non-communicating* (obstruction within the ventricular system). There are several causes of hydrocephalus during the first few months of life.

Congenital
Stenosis of the aqueduct accounts for 70 per cent of congenital causes. Others include: 'forking' (in which the aqueduct is replaced by two narrow channels); gliosis (an overgrowth of the subependymal neuroglia); absent or obstructed ventricular foraminae; the Dandy Walker syndrome (posterior fossa cyst, hypoplasia cerebellar vermis and hydrocephalus); or congenital absence of arachnoid granulations (see Wright, 1994).

Intraventricular haemorrhage
The microvasculature of the germinal matrix (an area of neuronal development that disappears by term) has an abundant arteriolar supply but is very fragile. Intraventricular haemorrhage (IVH) results from rupture of the microvasculature into the cerebral ventricles. The incidence correlates with the degree of prematurity (20 per cent of babies born weighing less than 1500 g are affected) and the clinical history of the baby. The aetiology of IVH is multifactorial. Sick or immature babies may have impaired or limited autoregulation, allowing changes in arterial blood pressure (e.g. in response to clinical procedures) directly to affect cerebral blood flow or volume. Arterial blood flow to the brain is further increased by hypercarbia, hypoxia or increased local metabolism (e.g. during seizures). Rupture of the micro-

vasculature may also be produced by rises in central venous pressure (e.g. high airway pressure, poorly synchronized mechanical ventilation, rapid infusion of intravenous fluid, patent ductus or pneumothorax). The risk of IVH is probably greater if coagulation is abnormal (see Hatch *et al.*, 1995; Roland and Hill, 1997).

Blood clot and debris from IVH can obstruct the aqueduct between the third and fourth ventricles or plug the arachnoid villi, impairing absorption of CSF. Blood may also cause obliterative arachnoiditis in the posterior fossa, obstructing the foraminae of the fourth ventricle. Hydrocephalus after a major bleed usually develops over a few days (see Roland and Hill, 1997).

Meningitis

Purulent meningitis can cause hydrocephalus by obstructing absorption of CSF by the arachnoid villi.

Spina bifida

Spina bifida is usually associated with the Arnold–Chiari malformation, in which the medulla and the inferior vermis of the cerebellum herniate into the cervical region of the spinal canal. The flow of CSF is impaired because the foraminae of the fourth ventricle are obstructed by adhesions. The aqueduct between the third and fourth ventricles may also be abnormal (see Wright, 1994).

The signs of hydrocephalus in a baby are (Wright, 1994):

a. A large head
b. Bulging fontanelles
c. The 'setting sun' appearance of the eyes, in which the eyeball seems to be depressed, revealing the sclera above the iris
d. Cranial nerve palsies (e.g. of the sixth, producing paresis of the lateral rectus; or the tenth, producing partial vocal cord paresis and stridor)
e. Retinal haemorrhages.

Papilloedema is uncommon in congenital, non-communicating hydrocephalus, because CSF pressure within the subarachnoid space of the orbital part of the optic sheath is not raised (Wright, 1995).

Hydrocephalus in babies is often well tolerated initially if the rate of rise of intracranial pressure (ICP) is slow, because:

a. The brain contains a lot of water, has fewer myelinated fibres and a large subarachnoid space, and is relatively compliant
b. The cranium can expand to accommodate the increased volume of CSF because the cranial sutures and fontanelles are not fused.

If the volume of CSF or other intracranial contents expands rapidly, ICP will rise because the dura is relatively stiff and cannot distend acutely.

Features in a baby suggesting decompensation of intracranial hypertension include: apnoea; poor feeding and vomiting; distension of scalp veins; irritability or coma; spasticity; bradycardia and hypertension; and seizures (see Tasker *et al.*, 1995).

2. For the anaesthetic plan, the following must be considered:

a. The general principles of anaesthesia for any small baby
b. The implications of prematurity
c. The problems associated with raised intracranial pressure (ICP)
d. Any complications of the operation.

Principles of anaesthesia

This baby should be managed in a hospital with adequate facilities and trained staff. In planning the anaesthetic technique, the basic principles of anaesthesia for a baby (e.g. use of appropriate equipment; the differences in physiology and pharmacology; the risks of hypothermia etc.) should be carefully considered.

Implications of prematurity

The associations of prematurity in this baby (now 43 weeks postconception) include: significant pulmonary disease (e.g. bronchopulmonary dysplasia or oxygen dependency); an increased risk of postoperative apnoea (Welborn, 1992); difficult venous access; subglottic stenosis and tracheomalacia; and anaemia. The baby may also have significant congenital abnormalities that of themselves are associated with premature birth (e.g. congenital heart disease, tracheo-oesophageal fistula etc.). Premature babies may be given a variety of medications. Diuretics are used in heart failure or bronchopulmonary dysplasia and may produce electrolyte disturbances, particularly hypokalaemia. Steroids are used in bronchopulmonary dysplasia and occasionally cause hypertension or glucose intolerance. Theophyllines stimulate breathing and are prescribed for apnoea and bradycardia of

Table 32.1 Medical management of post-haemorrhagic hydrocephalus (modified from Roland and Hill, 1997)

Medication	Mechanism of action	Major side effects
Acetazolamide	Carbonic anhydrase inhibitor, decreases CSF production by 50 per cent	Metabolic acidosis, nephrocalcinosis (if used with frusemide), potential toxic effect on myelin
Frusemide	Carbonic anhydrase inhibitor, decreases CSF production	Metabolic acidosis, dehydration, hypercalcaemia, hypercalcuria, possible toxic effect on myelin
Isosorbide	Osmotic agent, increased serum, decreased CSF formation	Hypernatraemia, diarrhoea and vomiting

CSF, cerebrospinal fluid.

prematurity. The therapeutic index is low; they can produce hyponatraemia and, in toxic plasma concentrations, cause fits, tachycardia, tremor or vomiting.

Problems of raised ICP
The main problems associated with hydrocephalus are the effects of its medical treatment (Table 32.1) and the risks of sudden cerebral decompensation during the induction of anaesthesia if the ICP is raised.

Complications of the operations
Haemodynamic instability may be seen when the surgeon decompresses the ventricles or inserts the drain. Very occasionally, excessive bleeding can occur if epidural veins are damaged.

Most babies with hydrocephalus are about 2 kg or more when a drain is inserted, because the complications of the procedure in smaller babies are unacceptably high. Shunts are not inserted immediately after IVH because the CSF remains very viscous after a bleed and does not drain well (Mackersie, 1989).

During the preoperative assessment, the anaesthetist must look carefully for the signs and symptoms of intracranial hypertension and any problems associated with premature birth (see above). Questions should be asked regarding other perinatal problems (e.g. birth asphyxia) and postnatal history (e.g. duration of mechanical ventilation; repeated intubation of the trachea etc.). The baby must be weighed.

Plasma urea and electrolyte concentrations should be requested because of possible disturbances associated with medication (e.g. for hydrocephalus, heart failure or bronchopulmonary dysplasia) or poor fluid intake because of poor feeding or vomiting. Hypercalcaemia may need to be corrected before surgery because of the risk of asystole. Chronic hypernatraemia should be treated cautiously; a sudden reduction in plasma concentration may produce cerebral oedema and worsen intracranial hypertension. Hypoglycaemia significantly increases cerebral blood flow in new-born premature babies, and should be treated. The haemoglobin concentration must also be known; anaemia is associated with a greater risk of postoperative apnoea (Welborn, 1992) and increases cerebral blood flow (Roland and Hill, 1997). Blood loss is usually minimal during surgery, but blood should be cross-matched in case the enlarged epidural veins are damaged.

Sedative premedication is unnecessary and may depress ventilation and worsen intracranial hypertension or delay recovery. Topical anaesthetics such as eutectic mixtures of local anaesthetics (EMLA) or amethocaine (Ametop) reduce pain on insertion of intravenous cannulae. The systemic uptake of topical anaesthetics depends upon the maturity and integrity of the skin. The stratum corneum develops over the first few days of life, and maturity is a function of postnatal, rather than post-conceptional, age. EMLA can be safely used in infants of 3–12 months who are not taking methaemoglobin-inducing agents if the dose is limited to 2 g over 16 cm^2 for less than 4 hours (although it is not licensed in the UK for babies younger than 12 months). Ametop is licensed for use in babies as young as 4 weeks. Some anaesthetists prescribe atropine (20 μg/kg orally) to reduce airway secretions and the vagal effects on the heart. Others prefer to give it at induction of anaesthesia or to treat bradycardia.

The baby's cardiovascular, ventilatory and neurological status should be monitored carefully and frequently whilst awaiting surgery. A modification of the Glasgow coma score used for babies and children younger than 4 years of age is given in Table 32.2. If necessary, the ICP can be reduced before surgery by removing CSF by a ventricular tap through the anterior fontanelle (non-communicating hydrocephalus) or lumbar puncture (communicating hydrocephalus) under local anaesthetic (see Wright, 1994).

Babies with open fontanelles and unfused sutures can compensate for gradual increases in intracranial volume by expanding the cranium, but if the increase is sudden, ICP will rise because the dura is relatively non-compliant and cannot distend acutely.

Table 32.2 The Glasgow coma scale modified for use in babies and children younger than 4 years of age

Eyes:
- Open spontaneously   4
- React to speech   3
- React to pain   2
- No response   1

Best motor response:
- Spontaneous or obeys verbal command   6
- Localizes pain   5
- Withdraws from pain   4
- Abnormal flexion to pain (decorticate posture)   3
- Abnormal extension to pain (decerebrate posture)   2
- No response   1

Best verbal response:
- Smiles, orientated to sounds, follows objects, interacts   5
- Cries, but consolable; interacts appropriately   4
- Cries, inconsistently consolable; moaning   3
- Inconsolable, irritable   2
- No response   1

Acute increases in blood volume will result from high concentrations of inhalational anaesthetic agents, hypertension (if auto-regulation is disturbed), hypoxia, hypercarbia or high airway inflation pressures. ICP is also raised by attempted intubation in an awake or inadequately anaesthetized baby. The rise is not entirely explained by changes in arterial blood pressure, but can be prevented by intubating after muscle relaxation and anaesthesia. Intravenous induction of anaesthesia is probably the technique of choice, using an intravenous induction agent, a muscle relaxant to facilitate intubation and a small dose of a short-acting opioid such as alfentanil (5–10 μg/ml) or intravenous lignocaine (1 mg/kg) to attenuate the haemodynamic response to intubation. Larger doses or longer-acting opioids should be avoided because of the risks of ventilatory depression after surgery. Venous access can be difficult to obtain in babies born prematurely, and it may be necessary to look for veins on the scalp, chest or abdominal wall. An inhalational induction should be used very cautiously because of the vasodilatory effects on the cerebral circulation.

The objectives during anaesthesia are to avoid hypoxia, maintain a low normal end-tidal CO_2, and avoid reductions or increases in systemic blood pressure. To control carbon dioxide tension, the trachea must be intubated and the lungs ventilated. A baby with an enlarged cranium will have a large occiput, and this may make intubation difficult because of a greater tendency to flex the neck when supine. The baby's position for intubation can be improved by placing a thick layer of padding underneath the back, allowing the head to lie in the neutral position. The tube should be secured very carefully and it is important to ensure that both lungs are being ventilated, especially when the baby is finally positioned for surgery, because access to the head is limited once the surgeon starts. The large surface area of the head also increases the risk of hypothermia. Heat loss during the induction of anaesthesia can be minimized with an overhead heater in addition to using other methods to keep the baby warm. Excessive heat loss may continue during surgery because of the large radiant and evaporative surface.

The haemodynamic response to surgical incision can be reduced by infiltrating the scalp with local anaesthetic (e.g. bupivacaine 2 mg/kg). This will also provide postoperative analgesia. Blood loss is usually minimal, but is difficult to measure because it is mixed with CSF. Blood loss can be further reduced by infiltrating the skin with adrenaline (maximum of 5 μg/kg). Haemodynamic instability can occur during the operation: if the intracranial and arterial pressures are high, hypotension is sometimes seen when the ventricles are drained; and bradycardias and other arrhythmias may occur when the catheter is inserted, probably because of shifts within the brain (Steward, 1995).

At the end of the procedure, the muscle relaxant should be antagonized and the baby extubated only when he is vigorous and awake.

3. The baby should be cared for on a high-dependency unit after surgery because of the risks of postoperative apnoea in babies born prematurely and neurological deterioration if the shunt obstructs. The baby should be observed for a minimum of 12 hours free of apnoea before discharge to an ordinary ward. The nurses should monitor neurological status and oxygen saturation, breathing and heart rates continuously. The alarm limits should be set at an oxygen saturation of 90 per cent, apnoea interval of 15 s, and heart rate of 100 beats per minute.

Postoperative pain can be treated with infiltration with local anaesthetic at the time of operation and regular paracetamol 15 mg/kg 6-hourly afterwards.

Key learning points

- Non-communicating hydrocephalus with impaired absorption of CSF is more common than excessive secretion or communicating hydrocephalus.
- Anaesthesia follows general principles of neonatal anaesthesia, but the implications of prematurity, raised intracranial pressure and surgical complications affect technique.
- High-dependency or intensive care is needed after surgery.

Further reading

CONRAN, A. M. and KAHANA, M. (1998). Anesthetic considerations in neonatal neurosurgical patients. *Neurosurg. Clin. North Am.*, **9**, 181–5.

HATCH, D., SUMNER, E., HELLMANN, J. *et al.* (1995). Neonatal anaesthesia – specific conditions. In: *The Surgical Neonate: Anaesthesia and Intensive Care*. Ch. 4, pp. 148–209. Edward Arnold.

MACKERSIE, A. (1989). Anaesthesia for neurosurgery in paediatrics. In: *Textbook of Paediatric Anaesthetic Practice* (E. Sumner and D. J. Hatch, eds), Ch. 16, pp. 377–402. Balliere Tindall.

ROLAND, E. H. and HILL, A. (1997). Intraventricular hemorrhage and posthemorrhagic hydrocephalus. *Clin. Perinatol.*, **24**, 589–605.

STEWARD, D. J. (1995). Neurosurgery. In: *Manual of Paediatric Anesthesia*. Ch. 8, pp. 189–212. Churchill Livingstone.

TASKER, R. C., DEAN, J. M., ROGERS, M. C. *et al.* (1995). Reye syndrome and Reye-like illnesses. In: *Handbook of Pediatric Intensive Care* (M. C. Rogers and M. A. Helfaer, eds), Ch. 12, pp. 350–76. Williams & Wilkins.

WELBORN, L. G. (1992). Postoperative apnoea in the former preterm infant: a review. *Paed. Anaesth.*, **2**, 37–44.

WRIGHT, V. M. (1994). Hydrocephalus. In: *Surgery of the Newborn* (N. V. Freeman, D. M. Burge, M. Griffiths *et al.*, eds), Ch. 47, pp. 587–96. Churchill Livingstone.

Case 33

An 8-year-old boy having a femoral osteotomy develops widespread erythema and severe bronchospasm 40 minutes after the start of surgery and 60 minutes after your last intravenous injection. He is receiving an intravenous infusion of saline 0.45% and glucose 5%. He was born with a meningomyelocoele and had a ventriculo-peritoneal shunt inserted at 6 weeks of age for hydrocephalus. He has had numerous previous operations without problems, and has no known allergies.

Questions

1. What is the likely diagnosis? Describe the associated clinical features.
2. Describe the immediate treatment.
3. List the investigations.
4. What advice should be given for further surgical and anaesthetic management?

Answers

1. This is an anaphylactoid reaction. Anaphylactoid reactions to parenteral drugs begin up to 15 minutes after administration and worsen over 5–10 minutes (see Kam *et al.*, 1997), but here the onset of symptoms is late, suggesting absorption of the causal agent across the skin or wound. The most likely cause is latex, which typically causes symptoms 30–60 minutes after the start of the operation. Other clinical signs indicating an anaphylactoid reaction include: hypotension, tachycardia and cardiovascular collapse; angio-oedema, particularly around the eyes and mouth; urticaria or skin rash; and stridor.

   This boy has a 'high risk' for developing allergy to latex because he was born with a meningomyelocoele. Up to 70 per cent of children with spina bifida have IgE antibodies to latex proteins, and the risk of developing allergy to latex is 500 times greater than in children without spina bifida. Sensitivity is thought to occur because of recurrent exposure to latex through repeated catheterization of the bladder, multiple operations, disimpaction of the bowel (see Steiner and Schwager, 1995) and the insertion of ventriculo-peritoneal shunts.

   Other children at greater risk of allergy to latex include:

   a. Those having multiple operations
   b. Those with a history of imperforate anus, VATER syndrome or tracheo-oesophageal fistula
   c. Those with multiple allergies, atopy or unexplained previous anaphylactoid reaction during surgery (see Landwehr and Boguniewicz, 1996; Kam *et al.*, 1997)
   d. Those with urinary tract abnormalities requiring recurrent surgery or catheterization (Holzman, 1997; Dakin and Yentis, 1998)

e. Those with ventriculo-peritoneal shunts (despite absence of latex in the shunt) and/or cerebral palsy
f. Those with spinal cord injury.

Cross-reactivity can occur with certain fruits, e.g. banana, avocado, chestnut, passion and kiwi fruits (see Steiner and Schwager, 1995).

Anaphylactoid reactions to latex are caused by a type 1 (immediate hypersensitivity) reaction. Latex proteins cross-link with IgE on mast cells and basophils, leading to degranu-lation and release of the mediators of the clinical response – e.g. histamine, leukotrienes and prostaglandins (Holzman, 1993; Landwehr and Boguniewicz, 1996; Kam *et al.*, 1997; Dakin and Yentis, 1998).

2. The immediate treatment of a severe allergic reaction is to assess and treat problems identified in the airway, with breath-ing and with the circulation. Further management of latex allergy is as for any anaphylactoid reaction (Table 33.1; Association of Anaesthetists of Great Britain and Ireland and the British Society of Allergy and Clinical Immunology, 1995). In severe reactions adrenaline should be given early and may be required in large doses.

3. Investigation of the reaction should be delayed until the immediate problem has been adequately treated. The history provides the most important clues to diagnosis and details of events; timing of drug administration and signs and symptoms must be recorded carefully. Although the most likely diagnosis in this boy is latex allergy, reactions to other agents (e.g. anaes-thetic drugs, antibiotics, intravenous colloids etc.) must be excluded. For latex, clinical history in combination with total serum IgE is a more sensitive and specific predictor for patients at risk of anaphylaxis than specific testing because so many different latex antigen proteins exist and it can be difficult to obtain the correct type for testing. The Association of Anaes-thetists of Great Britain and Ireland and the British Society of Allergy and Clinical Immunology have made recom-mendations for the investigation of patients who have an anaphylactoid reaction during anaesthesia (Association of Anaesthetists of Great Britain and Ireland and British Society of Allergy and Clinical Immunology, 1995), including measur-ing a serum tryptase concentration and subsequent skin testing.

Table 33.1 Management of a patient with suspected anaphylaxis during anaesthesia (modified for children from the recommendations of the Association of Anaesthetists of Great Britain and Ireland and the British Society of Allergy and Clinical Immunology, 1995)

Initial therapy

1. Stop administration of agents likely to have caused the anaphylaxis
2. Maintain airway: give 100 per cent oxygen
3. Lay patient flat with feet elevated
4. Give adrenaline:
   - intramuscularly, 10 μg/kg repeated every 10 min according to the arterial pressure and heart rate until improvement occurs
   - intravenously, 1 μg/kg over 1 min for hypotension, with titration of further doses as required
   - in a patient with cardiovascular collapse, intravenous adrenaline 10 μg/kg at a rate of 1–2 μg/kg per min may be required until an adequate response has been obtained
5. Start intravascular volume expansion with suitable crystalloid or colloid (10 ml/kg)

Secondary therapy

1. Antihistamines – chlorpheniramine 0.2–0.4 mg/kg i.v. slowly, consider H_2 antagonists
2. Corticosteroids – hydrocortisone 4 mg/kg i.v.
3. Catecholamine infusion:
   - adrenaline, 0.05–0.1 μg/kg per min
   - noradrenaline, 0.05–0.1 μg/kg per min
   - isoprenaline, 0.05–1.0 μg/kg per min
4. Measure arterial blood gases and consider i.v. bicarbonate 0.5–1.0 mmol/kg for acidosis
5. Evaluate the airway before extubation
6. Bronchodilators may be required for persistent bronchospasm

Investigations

1. Do not undertake investigations until the immediate treatment of the emergency has been completed
2. Diagnosis is made on clinical grounds. It is important to make a detailed written record of events, including timing of administration of all drugs in relation to onset of reaction
3. Approximately 1 hour after the onset of the reaction, take 10 ml of venous blood into a plain glass tube; separate serum and store at $-20\,°C$ until it can be sent to a reference laboratory for measurement of serum tryptase concentration
4. The patient, his or her parents and the general practitioner should be made aware of the reaction and its implications

Concentration of serum tryptase

A rise in serum tryptase within 4 hours of the reaction confirms mast cell degranulation, but does not indicate the cause. Ten millilitres of venous blood should be put in a plain bottle, centrifuged to separate the serum, and the serum subsequently stored at $-20\,°C$ until the enzyme can be assayed.

Skin testing

Skin prick testing is reasonably sensitive and specific and, although less sensitive than intradermal testing, has a smaller incidence of anaphylactic reaction (see Holzman, 1993). Facilities for resuscitation and management of anaphylaxis should be available.

Skin testing is delayed by 4–6 weeks after the event to allow the concentrations of mediators to fall and immunoglobulin E to increase to normal concentrations. Patients should not be taking antihistamines or steroids, because these may modulate responses.

Drugs are prick-tested neat and in dilutions of 1 : 10. The solutions are applied to the skin and 'pricked' through the skin without causing bleeding. The sites are examined after 15 minutes for a wheal and flare reaction, and responses are compared with a positive control (histamine) and a negative control (phenol in saline) (Association of Anaesthetists of Great Britain and Ireland and British Society of Allergy and Clinical Immunology, 1995). Skin prick testing for latex has almost 100 per cent sensitivity and specificity (see Steiner and Schwager, 1995), but because numerous different latex proteins exist (see Holzman, 1993), samples of any suspected latex allergy triggers should be used for testing to ensure the sensitivity and specificity of the test (see Dakin and Yentis, 1998).

Other tests

Other tests include radio-allergo-absorbent tests (RAST), enzyme-linked assays (ELISA) and Western blot tests (see Holzman, 1993; Steiner and Schwager, 1995; Kam *et al.*, 1997). *In vitro* tests to identify antigen-specific immunoglobulin E are safer than intradermal testing. However, these tests identify only 50–87 per cent of patients with IgE sensitivity, and are not predictive of an anaphylactoid reaction actually occurring on exposure to latex.

Table 33.2 The latex allergy protocol developed at the Chelsea and Westminster Hospital, London (Dakin and Yentis, 1998)

IDENTIFICATION OF AT-RISK GROUPS:

1. History of anaphylaxis to latex or a positive skin prick test to latex
2. History of allergy/sensitivity to latex:
   - itching, swelling or redness after contact with rubber products
   - swelling of the tongue or lips after dental examination or blowing up balloons
3. High-risk groups without a history of latex sensitivity:
   - patients subject to repeated catheterization (e.g. spina bifida, urogenital abnormalities)
   - those who have undergone multiple surgical procedures
   - those with atopy/multiple allergies (especially fruit)

LATEX-FREE ENVIRONMENT FOR GROUPS 1 AND 2

NO SPECIAL PRECAUTIONS, BUT A HIGH INDEX OF SUSPICION FOR GROUP 3

General advice:

1. Ensure full awareness of all staff involved with the patient
2. Ideally, the patient should be in a side room with a designated nurse and signs declaring latex-sensitive patient
3. Keep numbers of people involved to a minimum
4. Trolley mattress must be covered completely with cotton sheeting

Peroperatively:

1. Premedication: ideally 24 hours preoperatively, with a minimum of two doses, and for at least 12 hours postoperatively. The issue of premedication is controversial – premedication is not as effective as avoiding the allergen. The suggested scheme is:
   - i.v. chlorpheniramine: 1–12 months, 250 μg/kg; 1–5 years, 2.5–5 mg; 6–12 years, 5–10 mg
   - i.v. ranitidine, 1 mg/kg
   - i.v. hydrocortisone, 2 mg/kg,
   - inhaled/nebulized inhalers for asthmatics
2. Put patient first on the operating list (or use a theatre unoccupied for at least 2 hours to significantly reduce the level of latex antigen in the atmosphere)
3. Remove all latex-containing items and substitute appropriate latex-free equipment
4. Place clear, visible signs on theatre doors
5. Induce anaesthesia in the operating theatre
6. Ensure there is no direct contact of the patient with latex – cover mattress, supports etc., and cover limbs with stockinette prior to use of tourniquets
7. Do not inject through or draw up through rubber bungs
8. Draw up all drugs, including emergency drugs, in latex-free syringes

continued on facing page

VIGILANCE

ENSURE LATEX-FREE ENVIRONMENT CONTINUES IN RECOVERY AND ON
THE POSTOPERATIVE WARD

LATEX-FREE BOX

1. Located in the main operating department, containing:
   - database of latex-free equipment
   - database of latex-containing equipment to be avoided
   - database of latex-containing equipment that can be used with
     modification
   - appropriate replacement of latex-free equipment
   - latex-free gloves are the single most important precaution

---

4. Children with clinical evidence of allergy to latex (e.g. allergy to
   balloons or rubber gloves, previous intraoperative reaction
   suggestive of latex allergy etc.), even without positive con-
   firmatory tests, should avoid any further exposure to latex.
   A careful history and awareness of those groups of children
   at greatest risk (e.g. spina bifida; genito-urinary surgery etc.)
   is thought to be the best method of identifying children most
   likely to develop anaphylaxis (see Dakin and Yentis, 1998).
   Organizations in some countries (e.g. the American College
   of Allergy and Immunology) recommend avoiding latex in
   children with spina bifida from the outset, and this advice
   could be extended to children with any recognized risk factor.
      The most important factor in preventing a subsequent
   reaction is to avoid exposure to latex. These precautions
   must continue postoperatively. Latex proteins are present in
   a bewildering number of medical products, and the term
   'hypoallergenic' does not exclude them. It is difficult to obtain
   information about products urgently. Some authors suggest
   establishing protocols for managing patients with latex allergy,
   and keeping a box of latex-free equipment available in theatre
   (see Table 33.2; Steiner and Schwager, 1995; Dakin and Yentis,
   1998). Education of staff is also vital. It is possible to anticipate
   a rate of allergic reactions of 0.0–0.3 per cent with latex-safe
   protocol operating if errors are not made (Holzman, 1997).
      Surgical gloves are a common source of latex proteins, and
   the amount released seems to depend upon the manufacturing
   process used (Holzman, 1993; Landwehr and Boguniewicz,
   1996). Latex particles from gloves can form aerosols, particularly if the gloves have been dusted with powder, because
   latex proteins are adsorbed onto cornstarch. Airborne latex

can produce bronchospasm and airway oedema in susceptible individuals. Latex-free gloves offering the same protection against the transfer of viruses as standard latex (e.g. neoprene) are available, and are the single most important precaution in preventing anaphylaxis. Vinyl gloves are not suitable, because they are permeable to HIV and hepatitis B. Medical staff should wash their hands carefully before handling patients with latex allergy to ensure that any residual latex particles are removed.

Latex is present in many pieces of equipment, such as breathing circuits, re-breathing bags, ventilator bellows, rubber stoppers from multidose vials, syringe plungers, blood pressure cuffs, urinary catheters and surgical drains, etc. Dakin and Yentis (1998) have published lists of equipment currently available in the UK that can or cannot be used. If injection ports have to be included in fluid delivery systems, they should be taped over and not injected through. Whenever possible, single injection glass ampoules without rubber stoppers should be used. Drugs should not be reconstituted by injecting through rubber stoppers; the stopper should be removed before reconstitution and the drugs drawn up in latex-free syringes.

Some latex-containing equipment has to be used, but direct contact with the patient should be avoided – for example, by interposing a microbial filter between the patient and breathing circuit; covering the table with sheeting; isolating the blood pressure cuff from the patient with stockinette; covering the site of oxygen saturation monitor with 'Tegaderm' or a latex-free glove; and isolating ECG leads from the patient with latex-free tape etc.

Premedication to modulate the allergic response if triggered is recommended by some, particularly during major operations (Steiner and Schwager, 1995; Dakin and Yentis, 1998). Others argue that it may mask the early signs of an allergic reaction; children at risk of a reaction to latex have been safely anaesthetized without prophylactic premedication when latex was scrupulously avoided (Holzman, 1997). Premedication does not remove the need to avoid latex risk or the risk of a serious reaction, but is designed to reduce its severity. Prophylactic premedication usually consists of histamine 1 and 2 antagonists, corticosteroids and, sometimes, β agonists given 12–24 hours before surgery and continued for 24 hours afterwards. The regimen used at the Chelsea and Westminster Hospital has been modified for children in Table 32.2.

Appropriate dilutions of adrenaline should be available and given in a dose of 0.1 μg/kg i.v. if the early signs of anaphylaxis occur (Kam *et al.*, 1997).

Key learning points

- Latex allergy is now more frequently recognized, and at-risk groups have been defined in the last 10 years.
- A protocol for avoiding latex exposure should be followed for those at risk or with a suspicious history.
- An anaphylaxis protocol should be displayed wherever anaesthesia is given.

Further reading

ADVANCED PAEDIATRIC LIFE SUPPORT GROUP (APLS) (1997). *The Practical Approach*, 2nd edn, pp. 92–4. BMJ Publishing Group.

ASSOCIATION OF ANAESTHETISTS OF GREAT BRITAIN AND IRELAND AND BRITISH SOCIETY OF ALLERGY AND CLINICAL IMMUNOLOGY (1995). *Suspected Anaphylactic Reactions Associated with Anaesthesia*. Association of Anaesthetists of Great Britain and Ireland and British Society of Allergy and Clinical Immunology.

DAKIN, M. J. and YENTIS, S. M. (1998). Latex allergy: a strategy for management. *Anaesthesia*, **53,** 774–81.

HOLZMAN, R. S. (1993). Latex allergy: an emerging operating room problem. *Anesth. Analg.*, **76,** 635–41.

HOLZMAN, R. S. (1997). Clinical management of latex-allergic children. *Anesth. Analg.*, **85,** 529–33.

JOLLIFFE, D. M. (1999). Anaphylaxis. *Royal College of Anaesthetists Newsletter*, **45,** 59–62.

KAM, P. C. A., LEE, M. S. M. and THOMPSON, J. F. (1997). Latex allergy: an emerging clinical and occupational health problem. *Anaesthesia*, **52,** 570–75.

LANDWEHR, L. P. and BOGUNIEWICZ, M. (1996). Current perspectives on latex allergy. *J. Ped.*, **128,** 305–12.

STEINER, D. J. and SCHWAGER, R. G. (1995). Epidemiology, diagnosis, precautions, and policies of intraoperative anaphylaxis to latex. *J. Am. Coll. Surg.*, **180,** 754–61.

Case 34

A 4-year-old boy with a trisomy 21 and a heart murmur presents at the local dental hospital for outpatient dental extractions under general anaesthesia. He has had no previous operations.

148

Questions

1. What associated abnormalities are important to the management of anaesthesia?
2. What are the important points of preoperative assessment?
3. Describe the anaesthetic plan.

Answers

1. Trisomy 21 has several associations of importance to anaesthesia.

Learning difficulties
Children with trisomy 21 are generally amiable but have a variable degree of intellectual impairment. They may have a limited ability to understand procedures or cooperate with them.

Congenital heart disease
Congenital heart disease occurs in 26 per cent of these children (Table 34.1), usually producing a left-to-right shunt and increased pulmonary blood flow. Pulmonary vascular disease occurs earlier and more frequently compared with children without trisomy 21 but with similar cardiac abnormalities. This increased susceptibility may result from the high incidence of chronic hypoxia secondary to: obstructive and central sleep apnoea; recurrent pulmonary infections; or hypoventilation caused by muscle hypotonia.

Children with significant cardiac lesions tend to have corrective operations in early infancy before irreversible pulmonary hypertension develops. Surgical repair may produce conduction defects.

Pulmonary vascular disease can occur without congenital heart disease.

Table 34.1 Common cardiac defects in children with trisomy 21 (Kallen *et al.*, 1996)

Cardiac anomaly	Percentage of total cardiac anomalies
Endocardial cushion defects	39
Ventriculo-septal defects	28
Atrial septal defects	7
Patent ductus arteriosus	4
Tetralogy of Fallot	4

Abnormalities of the airway

Airway obstruction is common during anaesthesia. Contributing factors include a large tongue and small mandible, adeno-tonsillar hypertrophy, and a short, broad neck (see Mitchell *et al.*, 1995). Subglottic stenosis is reported in up to 6 per cent of patients. Although the incidence of congenital stenosis may be increased, more important factors are probably the frequency of tracheal intubation early in life because of major surgery and the use of too large a tube because of small body size for age. About one-quarter of children require tracheal tubes one or two sizes smaller than anticipated. Post-extubation stridor is common.

Obstructive sleep apnoea

Obstructive sleep apnoea is a syndrome of upper airway obstruc-tion, hypoventilation and oxygen desaturation during sleep (see Warwick and Mason, 1998). Obstructive sleep apnoea in otherwise normal children is usually associated with adeno-tonsillar hypertrophy. The syndrome is commonly associated with trisomy 21.

Severe and longstanding obstructive sleep apnoea produces chronic hypoxaemia, hypercarbia, insensitivity to carbon dioxide and a reliance on the hypoxic drive for breathing. Pulmonary hypertension secondary to hypoxic pulmonary vasoconstriction will cause right ventricular hypertrophy, and may result in pro-gressive right ventricular failure (cor pulmonale) (see Warwick and Mason, 1998).

Children with significant obstructive sleep apnoea syndrome are sensitive to anaesthetic agents, sedatives and opioids because these decrease the tone in the pharyngeal muscles and inhibit the arousal and ventilatory responses to hypoxia, hypercarbia and airway obstruction. This sensitivity persists into the postoperative period (Warwick and Mason, 1998). They may also present with acute heart failure or arrhythmias during anaesthesia.

Immune deficiency and recurrent respiratory tract infections

One-third of children with trisomy 21 presenting for routine surgery have a respiratory tract infection. Immunodeficiency increases susceptibility to all infections, particularly of the respira-tory tract (see Mitchell *et al.*, 1995).

Instability of the atlanto-axial joint

Trisomy 21 is associated with a generalized laxity of ligaments, including the transverse atlantal ligaments holding the odontoid process close to the anterior arch of the atlas. Between 10 and 15 per cent of children have radiological evidence of atlanto-axial instability (atlanto-dens interval equal to or greater than 4–5 mm), with the risk of subluxation of C1 on C2. Instability is greatest during flexion. The majority of the children with evidence of instability on X-ray have no neurological problems, but signs or symptoms occur in 1.5 per cent of all children with trisomy 21. Symptomatic subluxation after anaesthesia and surgery has been reported.

Small size for age
The majority of children with trisomy 21 are small for their ages; 47 per cent have weights below the fifth centile.

Muscle hypotonia
Muscle hypotonia occurs in the majority of these children and may impair ventilation and the child's ability to maintain an airway immediately after surgery (Mitchell *et al.*, 1995).

Other associations with trisomy 21 include hypothyroidism, epilepsy, leukaemia, and a high incidence of carrier status for hepatitis B (Mitchell *et al.*, 1995).

2. In addition to taking a history and making a routine physical assessment, the anaesthetist will need to determine the type and clinical effects of the cardiac abnormality and look for evidence of the important associations of trisomy 21.

Heart murmur
The most common heart abnormality is an endocardial cushion defect (Table 34.1), but these are usually corrected early in infancy before irreversible pulmonary hypertension develops. This boy has had no previous operations and, unless a more complex lesion has been missed, most likely has a small ventriculo-septal defect (VSD). Trisomy 21 can also be associated with tetralogy of Fallot. It is essential the anaesthetist knows the type of abnormality and its significance, and he or she should obtain the previous notes and may need to ask a cardiologist for an opinion depending upon the information available, the size and type of defect and the date of the last review. A child with a VSD who has been lost to follow-up may have developed significant and irreversible pulmonary hypertension (see below).

Most cardiac abnormalities associated with trisomy 21 produce a left-to-right shunt and do not cause cyanosis initially. Pulmonary hypertension occurs early and frequently. Echocardiography will help determine the anatomical abnormality, and can be used to assess ventricular function and shunt size and direction. Pulmonary hypertension is difficult to diagnose clinically; the murmur may become softer and shorter and the pulmonary artery appear enlarged on chest X-ray in late disease. The electro-cardiograph (ECG) is not very helpful. ECG evidence of right ventricular hypertrophy is another late sign and a poor indicator of disease (Bohn, 1998).

If the child is taking diuretics, concentrations of plasma urea and electrolytes should be requested. If he has cyanotic con-genital heart disease, his haemoglobin concentration must be measured. A high haemoglobin concentration is associated with a low-grade coagulopathy and thrombosis.

Obstructive sleep apnoea
The most common symptoms reported by parents of children with nocturnal sleep apnoea are snoring, noisy breathing, witnessed apnoea, restlessness, and frequent waking at night. Others include bed wetting, nightmares and headache in the morning. Adults with sleep apnoea syndrome tend to be obese and have somnolence during the day time, but in children poor weight gain, small size and hyperactivity are more characteristic (Warwick and Mason, 1998).

Investigations should aim to identify children with chronic hypoxia. A full blood count may show polycythaemia, and the ECG may give evidence of cor pulmonale (large P wave in leads II and VI, a large R wave in V1 and a deep S wave in V6). Other useful investigations include oxygen saturation monitoring during sleep, a chest X-ray to assess the size of the pulmonary artery, and echocardiography to determine ventricular size and function. Systemic hypertension can also occur (Warwick and Mason, 1998).

Respiratory tract infection
The anaesthetist should ask about productive cough and chronic nasal discharge and examine the chest for wheeze and signs of consolidation. A chest X-ray may be helpful.

Atlanto-axial instability and cervical cord compression
Preoperative X-rays are unreliable in predicting the risk of spinal cord damage under anaesthesia, and routine screening is prob-ably not helpful (Mitchell et al., 1995). Most anaesthetists do not request them. Children with trisomy 21 should probably have a comprehensive neurological assessment before and after

surgery in an attempt to identify patients with atlanto-axial sub-luxation. Signs and symptoms include neck pain, torticollis, head tilt, clumsiness, abnormal gait or falls, loss of bowel or bladder control, hyper-reflexia, clonus, extensor plantar reflexes, limb weakness or hemi-, para- or quadriplegia. Any child with symptoms should be referred to an orthopaedic or neuro-surgeon for further assessment.

3. A child with trisomy 21 has several potential risks associated with anaesthesia, and he should have his dental extractions in a hospital with the facilities to manage all his potential intra- and postoperative complications. If his cardiac abnormality is minor (e.g. a small VSD) and he is otherwise well, there is no contraindication to admission as a day patient. All the anaesthetist's explanations should be appropriate to the child's intellectual level.

If this boy has evidence of cor pulmonale secondary to obstructive sleep apnoea, the anaesthetist should consider delaying surgery until his condition has been improved with controlled oxygen, continuous positive airway pressure and diuretics, and any respiratory tract infection has been treated. Simple analgesics can be prescribed for pain, and antibiotics if there is evidence of dental infection. The dentist may wish to use a temporary dental dressing.

Children with cyanotic cardiac disease should not be deprived of fluid for too long because of the risks of thrombosis associated with polycythaemia. It may be wise to prescribe intravenous fluids before surgery if the haemoglobin concentration is greater than 15 g/dl.

Some children (e.g. those with tetralogy of Fallot, or the very anxious) will benefit from sedative premedication. Suitable drugs include: temazepam, 0.5 mg/kg; midazolam, 0.5 mg/kg; trimeprazine tartrate, 2 mg/kg. Sedation should be used cautiously if significant obstructive sleep apnoea is suspected. Topical anaesthesia with a eutectic mixture of local anaesthesia (EMLA) or amethocaine gel (Ametop) will reduce the pain of venous cannulation. Premedication with atropine may be useful to reduce airway secretions. An exaggerated cardiac and mydriatic response has been reported, but increased cardiac sensitivity has not been supported by subsequent studies (Mitchell et al., 1995).

Antibiotic prophylaxis against bacterial endocarditis must be given according to accepted guidelines (Table 34.2). The choice of induction of anaesthesia will depend upon the degree of

Table 34.2 Prevention of endocarditis in patients with a heart valve lesion, septal defect, patent ductus or prosthetic valve having dental procedures (British National Formulary 2000)

1. *Under local or no anaesthesia:*

   - Patients who have not received more than one dose of a penicillin in the previous month and have never had endocarditis – oral amoxycillin 3 g 1 hour before procedure; child < 5 years, 25 per cent of adult dose; child 5–10 years, 50 per cent adult dose

   - Patients with allergy to penicillin or who have received more than one dose of a penicillin in the previous month – oral clindamycin 600 mg 1 hour before procedure; child < 5 years, 25 per cent of adult dose; child 5–10 years, 50 per cent of adult dose

   - Patients who have had endocarditis – amoxycillin + gentamicin (as for general anaesthesia)

2. *Under general anaesthesia:*

   - Patients at no special risk (excluding those who have received more than one dose of a penicillin in the previous month) –
     EITHER i.v. amoxycillin 1 g at induction and oral amoxycillin 500 mg orally 6 hours later; child < 5 years, 25 per cent of adult dose; child 5–10 years, 50 per cent of adult dose
     OR oral amoxycillin 3 g 4 hours before procedure and 3 g as soon as possible after the procedure; child < 5 years, 25 per cent of adult dose; child 5–10 years, 50 per cent of adult dose
     OR oral amoxycillin 3 g + oral probenecid 1 g 4 hours before procedure

   - Patients at special risk (including those with a prosthetic valve or who have had endocarditis) – i.v. amoxycillin 1 g + i.v. gentamicin 120 mg at induction and oral amoxycillin 500 mg 6 hours later; child < 5 years, amoxycillin 25 per cent of adult dose and gentamicin 2 mg/kg; child 5–10 years, amoxycillin 50 per cent of adult dose and gentamicin 2 mg/kg

   - Patients with allergy to penicillin or who have received more than one dose of a penicillin in the previous month –
     EITHER i.v. vancomycin 1 g over at least 100 minutes + i.v. gentamicin 120 mg at induction or 15 minutes before the procedure; child < 10 years, vancomycin 20 mg/kg and gentamicin 2 mg/kg
     OR i.v. teicoplanin 400 mg over at least 100 minutes + i.v. gentamicin 120 mg at induction or 15 minutes before the procedure; child < 14 years, teicoplanin 6 mg/kg and gentamicin 2 mg/kg
     OR i.v. clindomycin 300 mg over at least 10 minutes at induction or 15 minutes before the procedure and oral or i.v. clindamycin 150 mg 6 hours later; child < 10 years, 25 per cent of adult dose; child 5–10 years, 50 per cent of adult dose

i.v. intravenous.

cooperation of the child, the complexity of the cardiac abnormality, and the ease of venous cannulation. All infusions and injections must be free of air because of the risk of paradoxical air embolus. The speed of induction with a volatile agent in a child with a left-to-right shunt is not significantly increased. Induction with intravenous agents should theoretically take longer, but in practice the effect is minimal. Ketamine is associated with cardiac stability, even in children with complex cardiac disease. Care should be taken to avoid excessive decreases in systemic vascular resistance if the shunt is large because it may reverse producing hypoxia, hypercarbia and acidosis.

The anaesthetist's decision about maintenance again depends upon the presence of clinically significant problems, particularly congenital heart disease. Delivering anaesthesia through a nasal mask is probably not appropriate because of the difficulties maintaining a patent airway. Alternatives are intubation of the trachea and either spontaneous or positive pressure ventilation of the lungs or using a laryngeal mask airway. Excessive movement of the neck should be avoided, particularly flexion, because of the potential risk of atlanto-axial subluxation.

Postoperative analgesia can be provided using a combination of nerve blocks, paracetamol and non-steroidal anti-inflammatory drugs. Opioids are not necessary unless required as part of a 'cardiac stable' anaesthetic technique.

These children must be supervised closely in the recovery ward, because they often become agitated and can be difficult to manage.

If there is evidence of sleep apnoea, they should be observed on a high-dependency unit with monitoring of oxygen saturation and heart and breathing rates. Continuous positive airway pressure with humidified oxygen through nasal prongs or a mask may be helpful.

Key learning points

- The most important associated abnormalities in children with trisomy 21 are cardiac, airway and atlanto-axial.
- Look carefully for history, symptoms or signs of obstructive sleep apnoea, cor pulmonale or occult chest infection.
- Postoperative high-dependency or intensive care may be needed even after a short anaesthetic and surgical procedure.

Further reading

BRITISH NATIONAL FORMULARY (2000). *Infections*, **39,** 247–311.

BOHN, D. (1998). Anomalies of the pulmonary valve and pulmonary circulation. In: *Pediatric Cardiac Anesthesia*, 3rd edn (C. Lake, ed.). Appleton & Lange.

KALLEN, B., MASTROIACOVO, P. and ROBERT, E. (1996). Major congenital malformations in Down Syndrome. *Am. J. Med. Genetics*, **65,** 160–6.

MITCHELL, V., HOWARD, R., FACER, E. *et al.* (1995). Down's syndrome and anaesthesia. *Paed. Anaesth.*, **5,** 379–84.

WARWICK, J. P. and MASON, D. G. (1998). Obstructive sleep apnoea syndrome in children. *Anaesthesia*, **53,** 571–9.

Index